Ketogenic Diet - Intermittent and Water Fasting 2019:

2 Books In 1 - How to Master Weight Loss With Tried-And-True Methods & Incredibly Effective Therapeutic Approaches.

Leanne Williams Liz Vogel

Jason Berg   Eric Fung

without direct written permission from the author or the publisher.

Under no circumstances will any blame or legal responsibility be held against the publisher, or author, for any damages, reparation, or monetary loss due to the information contained within this book. Either directly or indirectly.

Legal Notice:

This book is copyright protected. This book is only for personal use. You cannot amend, distribute, sell, use, quote or paraphrase any part, or the content within this book, without the consent of the author or publisher.

Disclaimer Notice:

Please note that the information contained within this document is for educational and entertainment purposes only. All effort has been executed to present accurate, up to date, and reliable, complete information. No warranties of any kind are declared or implied. Readers acknowledge that the author is not engaging in the rendering of legal, financial, medical, or professional advice. The content within this book derived from various sources. Please consult a licensed professional before attempting any techniques outlined in this book.

By reading this document, the reader agrees that under no circumstances is the author responsible for any losses, direct or indirect, which are incurred as a result of the use of the information contained within this document, including, but not limited to, — errors, omissions, or inaccuracies.

Ketogenic Diet - Intermittent and Water Fasting 2019

- You will gain weight if you do not eat breakfast
- Eating increases your metabolic rate
- Hunger is decreased by frequent eating
- Weight loss can be achieved with a lot of small meals
- The brain requires a steady supply of glucose
- It is healthy to snack and eat frequently
- Fasting makes your body go into starvation
- There is a minimum amount of protein that can be utilized for every meal
- You lose muscle when you undergo intermittent fasting
- It is unhealthy to carry out Intermittent Fasting
- You eat a lot while fasting intermittently

Chapter 10: Frequently Asked Questions

- Who can fast?
- How to know when to fast?
- How long can you water fast for without causing any harm?
- How frequently do I have to water fast?
- Is tea allowed during a water fast?
- What amount of weight is lost on a water fast?
- Is it possible for me to lose muscle?
- What is ketosis?
- What is the difference between juice fasting and water fasting?
- Can I do a juice fast instead?
- How many glasses of water should I drink daily?
- Can I be productive during a fast?
- Won't I gain back more weight after a fast since my rate of metabolism will reduce while I'm fasting and after the fast?
- Can IBS be cured by water fasting?
- Can kidney stones result from water fasting?
- Can ulcers result from water fasting?
- Is an enema advisable?

Conclusion

Reference

Ketogenic Diet and Intermittent Fasting Guidebook

Discover the Easy Method That Men, Women, and Even Beginners Are Using for Weight Loss With These Simple Metabolic Therapies in 2019

Leanne Williams Liz Vogel

Introduction

In many circumstances, you might think that it is entirely acceptable to be considered short, too tall, or even slim. Anything is better than being called fat. Your weight should be watched closely instead of being ignored. For this reason, it has become imperative for everyone to be aware of their diets and to live a healthy life. Aside from the gross disadvantages that come with being overweight as far as physical activities, it also poses adverse health conditions (e.g., heart disease and type 2 diabetes) that may lead to long term issues or death if not properly managed. These issues have led experts to come up with many weight-loss therapy ideas over the years.

Of all the treatments that people have attempted in their journey to be able to lose weight, the ketogenic diet has proven to be very useful when it comes to providing results. Besides its weight-loss benefits, there are numerous other health advantages attached to this therapy. These are the reasons why many doctors have been recommending it to their patients. What's even more impressive is the fact that this treatment, combined with another weight-loss method, known as intermittent fasting, can have more significant results.

In this eBook, will give you a rundown of everything that you will need to know about ketogenic dieting. You will find great ways to lose extra pounds, but more importantly, there are also tips on how to combine this technique with intermittent fasting. At the end of your journey, you are armed with the best ways to proceed with keto dieting and intermittent fasting, understand the dos and don'ts of these weight-loss methods and that you have started seeing positive results that will last.

Chapter 1: What is Ketogenic Dieting?

The word 'ketogenic' originated from 'ketones,' from which 'keto' is derived. Ketones are a small fuel molecule used as an alternative to providing sugar in the body when glucose (blood sugar) is short in supply. When you are low on carbs, your body goes through a metabolic state known as ketosis. Ketosis is characterized by a rise in the level of ketones in the system. Here you start burning glucose due to the lack of energy. Keto diets, unlike other low-carb diets, are centered on this macronutrient which supplies about 90% of the body's calories. Ketones are created from fats, and they provide energy to the whole body, particularly to the brain. The brain is the powerhouse of the human body, and it is always working. Even when you are asleep. However, it cannot run directly on fat, unless it gets converted into either glucose or ketones.

Whenever there is a drop in the level of insulin in your body, the amount of fat that your system burns spikes because the stored fats become more accessible and make it easier for your body to utilize them. It is a fact that burning fat is one of the easiest ways to shed a few pounds. This process is also beneficial for the body, in the sense that it gives you enough energy and reduces the number of times that you get hungry and helps you stay alert and focused throughout the day. When you are on a keto diet, your body begins to run on fat all day long, so it is perfect for getting your weight under your control since it burns fats 24/7.

Once you have decided to go on a keto diet, you should avoid too much protein because it can easily interfere with ketosis. That's why you need to employ some tricks, as well as a conscious effort, to get the results you desire. For instance, you must eat very low levels of carbohydrates in a day. Keep in mind that there are foods with extremely high levels of carbs, e.g., banana. There are about 27 grams of carbs in a medium sized banana. When you start on a keto diet, you should also remember that reaching ketosis does not take place overnight. Retraining your liver to produce ketones is not an easy feat. It typically takes a few days to get to this metabolic state.

In summary, the keto diet is a low-carbohydrate diet, which is used to burn fat more easily and quickly by allowing you to consume more fats than carbohydrates. It follows a dietary plan of about 60 to 70% fat, 15 to 30% protein, and 5 to 10% carbs (Perfect Keto, n.d.).

Generally, it is considered to be safe for almost everybody, but there are some groups of people to whom special consideration should be given. Those on medication for diabetes or hypertension, as well as mothers that are breastfeeding, should consult with their doctor before starting any diet or lifestyle changes.

History of Keto Diet

Fasting dates as far back as the twentieth century when ancient Greek physicians utilized it as a treatment for diseases like epilepsy and other health issues (Occhipinti, 2018). They also considered it an essential component of a healthy lifestyle. Ketogenic dieting is an eating pattern that birthed in the form of fasting to treat epilepsy in France in the year 1911. For over 2000 years this method has served as a standard practice across the world and is said to be the only treatment for epileptic patients that was recorded by Hippocrates. This is the first known use of the therapy before it was adopted to help people lose weight, which is now its most common use in the contemporary world.

According to a study, patients with epilepsy who took meals with low calories and tried fasting suffered from fewer seizures and less effect from the condition (Occhipinti, 2018). At first, the results from this routine were impressive, but as time passed, it was discovered that they were only temporary since the seizures returned in many patients as soon as they went back to their original diets. This led to doctors focusing their research on eliminating starch and sugars instead of placing an equal restriction on all calories. A particular point of reference is the case of Dr. Wilder of Mayo Clinic, (Occhipinti, 2018) who discovered that patients had fewer seizures when they ate high-fat and low-carb diets.

He created the ketogenic diet as a way of replicating the metabolism that would occur when fasting. Adopting this method kept the patients' bodies in a fasted state by requiring it to burn fat instead of glucose. This convinced the metabolic actions of the body to act as if it was starving, even though it was taking in enough calories and nutrition to sustain it and remain in a comfortable state. A few years later, this therapy became known as the standard keto diet, thanks to Dr. Peterman, another physician of the Mayo Clinic (D'Andrea Meira et al., 2019). In this approach, the fat-to-protein ratio is 4:1. There is a 90% distribution of calories from fat, 6% from protein, and just 4% from carbs. Even though this ratio is considered the standard, 3:1 is also beneficial. His proportions are still used today.

While fasting was useful for the treatment of epilepsy, the keto diet was found to be more sustainable with the same results as fasting (Land, 2018). Since this therapy has now run into its second century, the basic eating strategy has remained relatively unchanged. According to nutritionists, one gram of protein per kilogram of body weight should be consumed, while ten to fifteen grams of carbs should be taken daily (Patz, 2017). The rest should be filled with fat. Initially, doctors placed more emphasis on accurate measurements of foods for better results. Foods were weighed at the time before consumption to ensure that participants were kept on track.

In the 1990s, keto diets became unpopular as they merely served as objects of historical study rather than medical facts (Occhipinti, 2018). It, however, made a comeback in the year 1994, thanks to the TV show called Dateline. In a particular episode in October, a two-year-old boy named Charlie had a case of uncontrollable seizures until he was placed on the keto diet. On the show, viewers saw how the diet reduced Charlie's seizures, and this sparked an outbreak of interest and more scientific research about the method.

After it resurfaced, the keto diet was adopted as a viable option to treat epilepsy once again. It has also gained widespread acceptance and is now available at almost all children's hospitals. People show scientific interest in addition to the role that it plays in neurological disorders.

It is important to note; however, that a keto diet is not only good for just epilepsy. If it were, it would have been less famous since epilepsy isn't a common condition. The most typical use of the diet is for losing weight. Though it is not entirely clear when this diet has become accepted as a weight-loss medium, it is known that the early and late 90s has been dominated by the Atkins diet which shares the same perspective on carbs as the ketogenic diet. The renewed interest on the method made researchers pry into the possible effects that it can have on healthy humans, and the results are quite impressive. Today the keto diet has gained recognition that goes far beyond the mere treatment of epilepsy.

An Outline for the Keto Diet

There is no standard ratio for the measurement of the intake of essential nutrients (carbohydrate, protein, and fat) while someone is on a keto diet, but it sets the drastic cut in the consumption of carbs as its premise. Typically, the advisable ratio for your daily level of carbs should be reduced to 50 grams, which is less than the number of carbs found in a bagel. For better results, you can decrease it further to as low as 20 grams in a day. For a diet of 2000 calories, it is advisable for your meal plan to consist of 165 grams of fat, 75 grams of protein, and 40 grams of carbohydrates. While the level of protein in a keto diet is kept at a minimum ratio, it still provides enough nutrients to preserve body mass, as well as the muscle without preventing ketosis.

Although there are different versions of the ketogenic diet, the carbohydrate consumption is always kept at a minimum while the foods that are high in saturated fats get pushed to the forefront.

Here are the different diets to choose from.

Standard Ketogenic Diet

This diet consists of foods with high fat, moderate protein, and low carbs. The usual ratio is 75% fat, 20% protein, and 5% carbohydrate.

Clinical Ketogenic Diet

When you go through clinical keto dieting, you can expect intervals of high carb refills. This means that you have a few days while on the ketogenic diet and then take a break to consume a high amount of carbohydrates. For example, you decide to go on a five-day keto diet. Right after those five days, plan for a day when you will only eat a lot of starchy foods.

Targeted Ketogenic Diet

Here, when on a keto diet, you are allowed to add carbs around workouts.

High-Protein Ketogenic Diet

This version is similar to the standard keto diet, in the sense that you have to eat more protein than what is recommended. So if you consume 65% fat and 5% carbohydrate, you need 35% protein.

Nevertheless, you should take note that scientists have only been able to gather enough research on the standard ketogenic diet. Both the clinical and targeted keto diets are more often used by bodybuilders and athletes who need to keep their body in peak condition. For this reason, the focus will be more on a standard ketogenic diet in this eBook.

When on a ketogenic diet, it should be followed faithfully until you shed your desired amount of weight. After that, it is vital to keep up with your weight-loss goal by preventing yourself from gaining extra pounds. To ensure that you keep it off, you are expected to follow the diet for a few days or weeks per month.

The decision to switch to a ketogenic diet may seem overwhelming and complicated. It really doesn't have to, as long as you stick to the dos and don'ts. Reaching a state of ketosis is your primary goal. This is attained by eating a low intake of carbs, so remember that this can only be achieved when the body is deprived of starchy sources. While some individuals may get into a state of ketosis by cutting their carbohydrate level down to 20 grams, others may achieve the same result with a far higher amount of carb consumption. Generally, the lower the intake of carbs, the easier it is to reach and stay on ketosis. This is why it matters to eat keto-friendly foods, such as eggs, chicken, condiments, fatty fish, meat, full-fat dairy, full-fat cheese, nuts and seeds, nut butter, avocado, and other non-fatty vegetables.

The main foods to avoid are pastries (bread and other baked foods), sweets and sugary foods, sweetened beverages beans and legumes, pasta, grains, and grain products (e.g., wheat, rice, oats, and cereals). Starchy vegetables, high-carb sources, fruits, and some alcoholic drinks should also be avoided. Though it is essential to stay away from foods that provide carbohydrates, low-glycemic fruits like berries can be consumed in small amounts as long as you make sure that you are taking them in a macronutrient range. It also is essential to say no to processed foods and unhealthy fats such as margarine, shortening oils, and vegetable oils while sticking to good sources. The examples of processed foods that should be avoided include hot dogs, frozen meals, and fast food. Diet versions of foods that contain artificial colors, sweeteners, and alcohol should be avoided as well.

A One-Week Keto Menu

Just like any other new venture, you may find it quite challenging to come up with a perfect menu for your keto diet. Remember, even though this can be uncertain, it does not have to be complicated. The first thing to keep in mind when planning your meals is that everything you consume has to have more fat and fewer carbs. So, here is an example of a simple yet perfect menu for your one-week keto diet.

Sunday

Breakfast: Coconut milk chia pudding with coconut and walnuts on top.

Lunch: Cheese and turkey, avocado Cobb salad made with greens and hard-boiled eggs.

Dinner: Coconut chicken curry.

Monday

Breakfast: Two eggs with pasteurized butter and sautéed green vegetables.

Lunch: Bunless grass-fed burger with cheese, avocado, and mushrooms on top a bed of greens.

Dinner: Pork chops with green beans sautéed in coconut oil.

Tuesday

Breakfast: Mushroom Omelet.

Lunch: Tomato stuffed with tuna salad on top of a bed of greens with celery on the side.

Dinner: Grilled salmon with spinach sautéed in coconut oil.

Wednesday

Breakfast: Bell pepper stuffed with egg and cheese.

Lunch: Arugula salad with hard-boiled eggs, avocado, turkey, and blue cheese.

Dinner: Roast chicken in cream sauce with sautéed broccoli.

Thursday

Breakfast: Keto granola toppings on full-fat yogurt.

Lunch: Cauliflower rice steak bowl with cheese, salsa, herbs, and avocado.

Dinner: Bison steak with cheesy broccoli.

Friday

Breakfast: Baked avocado egg boats.

Lunch: Caesar salad with chicken.

Dinner: Pork chops with vegetables.

Saturday

Breakfast: Cauliflower toast with cheese and avocado toppings.

Lunch: Bunless salmon burgers with Pesto toppings.

Dinner: Zucchini noodles and meatballs with parmesan cheese.

As you can see in the above menu you can have different and nicely flavored meals, even when you are following a keto diet. Though most of these foods are based on animal products, the menu is also beneficial for vegetarians as there is a wide range of vegetables to choose from here. Recipes for all of these items can be found on the internet.

You may want to consider snack options from the extensive list of keto-friendly snacks available out there as well. Keep in mind that snacking between meals can help you keep hunger at bay and help you to stay on track.

Chapter 2: Side Effects of Ketogenic Diets

As mentioned earlier, even though the science behind it has not been proven yet, the keto diet has been a very potent remedy for cases of seizures in children with epilepsy. Francine Blinten, a certified nutritionist and public health consultant, who has used the diet on cancer patients with peculiar conditions, warns that the keto diet will do more harm than good, especially in people with kidney problems.

While there are a whole lot of gains such as weight loss and other health benefits when you go the ketogenic way, some experts frown at the diet, stating that there are more risks associated with a high level of fat (BMJ, 2016). According to a few of them, the diet is a total no-no when it comes to using it to lose weight due to the not-so-pleasant side effects that may occur with it. As well as its unsustainable nature. Other professionals who are in favor of the diet also agree that, if it isn't executed well, it might become disastrous to you while following the diet. So, if you intend to choose the keto technique to shed a few pounds, you may want to study the possible downsides that are connected to it.

The ketogenic diet is gradually taking precedence over all other weight-loss therapies. People across the globe who want to lose weight have embraced it as a way of burning fat in as few as ten days. Though the proponents of this diet say that it is an easy way to make the body burn its own fat through low-carb dieting and that it provides more energy to dieters, nutritional experts claim that it is not a safe method to lose body fat. While others believe that it is an easy way to enter starvation mode as the body merely loses water weight while on a keto diet. According to them, when the body enters into ketosis, it begins to lose muscle, leading you into a fatigued state, then eventually extreme hunger. Some folks refuse to back up this idea, but they say that they do not recommend the diet to someone who wants to gain muscle. The heart, after all, is also a muscle and is at risk when you subject yourself to a keto diet. This points to the fact that the weight-loss technique cannot be entirely safe for the muscles. Therefore, it is more advisable to try the ketogenic diet under the supervision of a clinical expert instead of doing it on your own for an extended period.

Here are some symptoms that going on a ketogenic diet can cause and you should consider before starting on this journey.

The Keto "Flu"

The keto flu is a combination of several physical indications that begin to manifest in someone who follows a ketogenic diet. While it is comprised of different symptoms, it feels like influenza. This is the result of the adaptation of the body to a new diet that consists of a little number of carbohydrates. As you may recall that in the keto diet, the body is forced to produce ketones, which are the byproducts of fat. Because of that, they replace glucose and become the primary source of energy. In normal circumstances, ketones are kept in reserve to provide power when simple sugar is not available. The switch takes place in rare cases of starvation or fasting. When the body begins to be deprived of carbohydrates during keto dieting, it reaches a state of ketosis. That is the time when the diet starts working. Due to this, you may not feel too well at first. This is when you might begin to suffer from the keto flu. The symptoms of this condition come in the form of vomiting, constipation, nausea, and irritability. You will also begin to urinate continually due to the high level of ketones produced by the body during the breaking down of fat. These ketones then get flushed out of your system through frequent and increased urination. The high rate of urination also leads to the uncontrollable loss of electrolytes, which then aggravates these symptoms. You will then be dehydrated and experience other indications of influenza, including dizziness, fatigue, and muscle soreness. The fact that carbohydrates are the significant sources of energy and stimulations makes you, who is short of it, crave sugar, experience brain fog, and have difficulty concentrating. It is similar to the signs of withdrawal.

Though the flu-like symptoms can range from mild to severe, they also vary from one to another. The signs typically start to manifest within the first few days of the diet and may last for about one week. In some people, though, the indications remain longer. They can also become causes of grief. Even to the extent that some dieters may use it as a sufficient reason to give up. The good news, however, is that there are ways to reduce the symptoms of keto flu. It is also important to note that the flu is not contagious, so there should absolutely be no cause for alarm.

Getting Rid of the Keto Flu

The symptoms of the ketogenic flu can stress you out since it may last for a week or more. You may also find it extremely challenging to adapt to the diet, but here are a few tips to help your system go through the transition phase more quickly.

Hydrate Yourself

For your general well-being, it is vital to stay hydrated. When you are trying to adopt the keto diet, you may want to consider drinking more water than you are used to, to allow your body to accept the new routine faster and reduce the symptoms of keto flu. When you try this diet, you shed water more efficiently. The reason for this is that glycogen, which is the stored form of carbohydrates, binds with water in the body. The glycogen levels are forced to drop with the reduction of dietary carbohydrates. Thus causing water to be excreted from the system. Hydration will help reduce symptoms like fatigue and muscle cramping. For this reason, it is imperative to replace fluids when you are experiencing diarrhea in association with keto flu since it can also cause an additional loss of bodily fluids.

Replace Electrolytes

If you are trying to tackle the keto flu, it is crucial to replace dietary electrolytes by getting adequate amounts of minerals that provide them.

Insulin is an essential hormone that absorbs glucose from the bloodstream. During the keto diet, the level of insulin decreases, causing the kidneys to release an excess quantity of sodium from the body. There are a lot of dietary restrictions that come with the ketogenic diet, especially when it comes to foods that are high in potassium, such as beans, fruits, and starchy vegetables. When your goal is to adopt this diet, you need to make up for these nutrients to be able to push through the entire journey. To acquire minerals, you should look for foods that are capable of maintaining a healthy balance of electrolytes. These can be avocados, leafy vegetables, and of course, salt. Not to mention higher levels of magnesium can help to reduce muscle cramps, headaches, and sleep issues.

Get Enough Sleep

In the early phase of the ketogenic diet, fatigue and irritability seem to be some of the major complaints that you might hear among individuals who are attempting to adapt to this regimen. The keto flu can worsen due to lack of sleep because it causes an increase in cortisol. Cortisol is a stress hormone that is released by the adrenal glands that affect your mood. If you are experiencing the keto flu, and are finding it difficult to sleep, here are some tips that may help:

1. Cut out ambient lights

When trying to doze off, lights are the most significant distractions. Luckily, it is easy to deliberately block them out by staying away from anything and everything that produces light. Draw the blinds, shut off your mobile phone, television, and computer in your bedroom to create a favorable environment for restful sleep.

2. Take a bath

Just before you get ready to go to sleep, make sure you relax your nerves and muscles by taking a shower or a bath. They are an effective way of calming every part of your body and feel refreshed. It is also a good idea to add Epsom salt or lavender oil to your bath water to help your system to wind down and relax as you prepare for bedtime.

3. Reduce your intake of caffeine

Not only is it a known fact that caffeinated drinks are addictive, but it is also important to note that they may affect your sleep by keeping you awake for longer hours than you typically want to. You should train yourself to stay away from caffeine in the early stages of the ketogenic diet or when you are suffering from the keto flu. If you must drink caffeinated beverages, make sure that you have them early in the day when you do not need to go to sleep. A good rule is to not have anything caffeinated after mid-day. This will guarantee that, by evening, you are finally ready to take that much-needed rest since the drink has undoubtedly worn off by that time.

4. Create a stable sleeping pattern and wake up early

It is easy for your body to get used to a particular routine if you have subjected yourself to it over a specific period. Following one specific sleeping and waking pattern will help your system shut down and wake up at times based on how you have programmed it to. This way, your sleep pattern will normalize, and you can boost the quality of your rest.

Stick to Less Strenuous Exercises

While exercises are absolutely beneficial for weight loss and overall well-being, it is also essential to stay away from activities that are capable of straining your muscles and the rest of your body. This is an especially useful tip for individuals who are experiencing the keto flu. Some of the symptoms that are common in the first week of the diet are stomach discomfort, fatigue, and muscle cramps. These are only a few reasons why you need to give an adequate amount of rest to your body during this phase. Even though activities like cycling, weightlifting, running, and other strenuous workouts may seem like a go-to when you are on your weight-loss journey, it is essential to shelve these exercises for the time being. You need to allow your system enough time to adapt to its new fuel sources. You can still exercise, but it is a better option to participate in activities such as yoga, leisure biking, and walking.

Eat Enough Fats and Transition Slowly

When introducing the keto diet to your body, it's essential to keep in mind that you will not be able to adopt the entire program all of a sudden. It is a good idea to take it slow. The first stage of the diet may force you to crave foods that are not part of the ketogenic plan, e.g., bread, pasta, bagels, and cookies. Seeing fat as the primary source of energy will reduce your cravings and give you a sense of satisfaction over time. If you have a hard time getting rid of carbohydrates, you should gradually eliminate them instead of staying away from them all at once. As you get rid of carbs little by little, you should substitute them with fat and protein to allow your body to have a smooth transition and decrease the symptoms of keto flu in the process.

Reduce the Risk of Kidney and Heart Damage

When on a ketogenic diet, you may be prone to acute kidney damage as a result of the loss of electrolytes such as potassium, magnesium, and sodium. This is caused by constant urination, which has the potential to lead to dehydration, lightheadedness, kidney injury, or kidney stones. Someone who follows this program can also be at risk of developing cardiac arrhythmia. The minerals that are lost when you urinate are essential to keep the heart beating regularly. Electrolyte deficiency can be detrimental to your health as it may result in irregular heartbeat, which may prove to be fatal.

According to research in the Journal of Child Neurology, 13 out of the 195 epileptic children who were placed on the keto diet developed kidney stones (Kim, 2017). It was, further noted, however, that those kids who were given potassium citrate were less prone to kidney stones than the others. For these reasons, experts have advised that those who wish to go with this dietary plan should speak to their healthcare practitioner if they have kidney-related concerns. If a man consumes a lot of meat (mainly processed ones when on a diet), for instance, he will be more susceptible to kidney stones and gout. Gout is a severe and excruciating metabolic disease that causes high levels of uric acid in the blood and joints, causing pain. After all, while a high intake of animal protein increases your calcium and uric acid levels, the combination of kidney stones and high uric acid cannot keep you away from gout. Generally, the ketogenic diet is not so friendly with people who have kidney diseases. In truth, they are usually placed on a strict, low-protein diet by their doctors. This regulation may not align with the low-carb, high-protein pattern that keto dieters may need to follow.

While the ketogenic diet relies on a high level of fat to burn calories, it is essential to know that certain types of fat are not healthy to some parts of the body. For instance, saturated fats and your heart are not friendly with each other. To maintain a healthy heart, you have to stay clear of foods like butter, cheese, and red meat. When shopping for groceries, you should try to read the labels so that you know if they contain ingredients that might bring you more chaos than calm health-wise. Things like hydrogenated oils (a.k.a. Trans fat) should be avoided as they are capable of increasing the low-density lipoproteins (LDL), which are commonly known as "bad" cholesterol in the body while reducing the high-density lipoproteins (HDL) or "good" cholesterol. According to the American Heart Association (n.d.), such fatty acids will heighten your chance of heart diseases and stroke probability. These issues should be taken into consideration when deciding on the quality of fats that you will consume. If you want to try the keto diet, you ought to eat more plant-based unsaturated fats, which have been proven to protect the heart. E.g., olive oil, avocado oil, nuts, and seeds. If your system is already high in cholesterol, you should consult your doctor before starting to follow this diet to avoid putting your well-being at a higher risk.

It is essential to note that experts have contrasting views on the subject of cardiovascular health while on the ketogenic diet. While some researches show that the program may decrease the possibility of having heart disease, as well as the number of saturated fats, others claim that it increases the cholesterol and triglyceride levels of the keto dieters.

Know the Risk of Yo-Yo Dieting

Even though ketogenic dieting began as a treatment for children who were suffering from epilepsy, it has now gained widespread acceptance among adults who are hoping to lose weight. Its fast-growing popularity is connected to the fact that the diet helps people shed a few pounds in as little as one month. According to a research in the American Journal of Clinical Nutrition, obese men who tried the modified version of the keto diet, which involved eating more protein and less carbohydrates, lost about 14 pounds in a month compared to the control group that followed a medium-carb diet and merely lost around 10 pounds (Thorpe, 2017).

The good news is that some professionals say that the individuals who are on the program can keep the weight off entirely if they stay on the diet for a long time. Nonetheless, such a feat is not usually easy to accomplish. When you lose weight during the keto diet, and then you go back to your original eating habits, the reduced pounds are bound to return in no time. Regaining the weight that you have already lost may lead to more negative eating habits. One example of that is called yo-yo dieting, which leads to an increase in abdominal fat accumulation and a higher risk of diabetes. It is essential to stick to a particular diet to achieve long-term success than just the plan itself. For people who have social engagements and are exposed continuously to carb cravings, keto seems to be restrictive and harsh. It becomes increasingly difficult for them to follow the diet for the long term. Once they begin to see positive results, they ditch the program and return to their regular routine. When you turn to yo-yo dieting, you start to hang between the advantages and disadvantages of losing and gaining weight. Hence, yo-yo dieting is also known as weight circling, and it becomes almost inevitable.

Simply put, yo-yo dieting is the pattern of losing weight, regaining the weight that was lost, and losing it again. It is risky, in the sense that it leads to an increased appetite, which can cause you to gain extra pounds over time. It can also lead to a high percentage of body fats and muscle loss. Fatty liver, diabetes, heart disease, and high blood pressure are some of the risks associated with this habit. Yo-yo dieting may not be as bad as weight gain, but it is certainly not as good as weight loss. While research has yet to prove whether being overweight is worse than this technique or not, it is clear that it is better to make small, beneficial, and permanent changes on your diet to promote a healthy lifestyle. Even if the reduction of fats may be slow, the long-term modifications will improve your life and may also prolong it. And there may be a noticeable improvement in your physical fitness as well.

There are other potential side effects of the keto diet. These can include fatigue, irregular menstrual cycles, constipation, bad breath, sleep issues, and decrease in bone density. Aside from that, the effect on blood cholesterol levels has not been thoroughly studied because of the difficulty of tracking dieters on a long-term basis to discover the lasting results of the dietary plan. Nutritionists are also concerned that the high intake of fats, which are considered unhealthy, can hurt someone's health in the long run. The short-term effect that is manifested by the diet, which comes in the form of weight loss, makes it quite challenging to monitor the data as it can be confusing. When an overweight person loses weight, the heart becomes healthier, and the risk of diabetes decreases. Obese people tend to end up with better blood lipids and glucose levels once they start to lose weight. Another disadvantage of the diet is the fact that it limits the number of certain vegetables, legumes, fruits, and grains, which are often considered "unhealthy" in this program. While folks avoid these foods, they miss out on some essential phytochemicals, fiber, vitamins, and minerals that can only be found in those forms. Nutrient deprivation bears significantly negative health impacts, including the increased potential of acquiring diseases and loss of bone mass. The craving for weight loss, which leads most people to go on keto diets, makes them prone to health deficiencies as well due to the low amount of whole foods that are supposed to keep you from contracting cardiovascular illnesses, Alzheimer's, cancer, osteoporosis, as well as type 2 diabetes. The standing question is: are people willing to risk their well-being for short-term goals such as losing weight?

Good Fats vs. Bad Fats: All You Should Know

When it comes to health and nutrition, fats do not have the same rave reviews that vitamins and other nutrients have that seem to reassure people. This may cause you to feel skeptical about relying on fats to lose weight, considering that it is generally perceived as something to be avoided. The truth is, while some fats are bad for your cardiovascular health and overall well-being, other types can be beneficial, and people are advised to imbibe them as part of their diets. So, instead of staying away from them, it is better to go for the good while ditching the bad. But there is no way to eat essential fats if you have no clue about the differences between the two.

While research on continues to evolve, there are a few facts worth talking about. Dietary fats, also known as fatty acids, are obtained from plants and animals. They have been linked to some not-so-pleasant effects on the heart, while others have been proven to have significant health benefits. Often, people tend to underrate the importance of fats in the body, even though their value is similar to that of proteins and carbohydrates when it comes to giving energy. After all, there are bodily functions that rely on fats. To be specific, some vitamins need them to be able to enter the bloodstream and provide nutrients to the body. If you are entirely devoid of fats, chances are, those vitamins may not be in your system as well. All the same, you should consume fatty sources in moderation because excess calories can make you gain weight. While all foods and oils have fats in them, the more dominant type will determine whether they are good or bad for your body.

Bad Fats

These fatty acids are considered to be harmful to your health as they expose you to more health risks. The two types of bad fats are saturated and trans fats. Most foods that contain such fats stay solid when they are kept at room temperature. Such as beef or pork fat, shortening, and margarine.

Saturated Fats

Saturated fats come from animal products, especially high-fat meats and dairy goods. They can also originate from dark chicken flesh and poultry skin, fatty cuts of meats from beef, pork, and lamb, tropical oils like coconut oil, palm oil, and cocoa butter, lard, as well as dairy foods like whole milk, butter, cheese, sour cream, and ice cream. The term "saturated fat" refers to hydrogen atoms, which surround individual carbon atoms. Fatty acids contain a chain of carbon atoms, binding as many hydrogen atoms as possible. This means that it is saturated with hydrogen.

When a diet is rich in saturated fats, it causes the cholesterol level to shoot up, thus tilting the balance towards a more harmful low-density lipoprotein (LDL) and causing blockages in the arteries and other parts of the body. For this reason, nutritionists advise that saturated fats should be reduced to below 10% of calories in a day (WHO, 2018). The intake of foods that are rich in such fatty acids will, therefore, increase the level of cholesterol and LDL in the blood.

For ages, doctors have blamed the consumption of high cholesterol to heart damage, but the idea is now being questioned by modern healthcare experts. A study conducted by Harvard University researchers (2019) suggests that high levels of cholesterol may not be as bad as they are presumed to be when it comes to maintaining a healthy heart. A meta-analysis of 21 subjects revealed that the evidence that could prove that saturated fats are the causes of heart diseases was not enough (Harvard Health Publishing, 2015). Various researchers have found that cardiovascular health risks can now be reduced by replacing saturated fats with polyunsaturated ones. While the reduction rate may be low, the difference can benefit someone's health superbly. We recommend that the HDL should be compared to your total cholesterol level, as well. When the ratio is high, the experts believe that it is associated with the increased resistance of insulin and heart problems. The research concludes that polyunsaturated fats like vegetable oils and high-fiber carbohydrates are the best ways to reduce the risk of cardiovascular diseases. It is important to note, however, that it is quite dangerous to replace saturated fats with highly processed carbohydrates because the result may be the opposite of what you are looking to accomplish.

Trans Fats

Trans fats cannot be produced naturally; they are industrially made. They are absolutely detrimental to your health, and they must be avoided at all costs. During production, they go through a process that adds hydrogenated vegetable oil to solidify them. These fats make people three times more susceptible to health risks (such as coronary heart disease and stroke) than other fats. The reason is that they increase the LDL cholesterol levels while increasing the HDL cholesterol levels. These fats have also been linked to inflammation of the body, which is also capable of leading to heart diseases, diabetes, and stroke.

Basically, trans fats are not crucial to human life as they do not promote good health in any way. According to the Harvard School of Public Health (2019), about 50,000 cases of fatal heart attacks each year have been associated with trans fat. It is related to an increased risk of developing type 2 diabetes as well. Because food companies find these fats cheap and easy to produce, can be used several times in commercial fryers and they have a long shelf-life and appealing taste, they have become more and more popular. These are a few of the reasons why trans fats are used in fast-food outlets and restaurants.

Some states in the United States have either already banned trans fat or are in the process of doing so. As a result of labeling laws, the manufacturers that make claims of no trans fats or zero grams of trans fat, still have hydrogenated oil content. It is, therefore, essential to read through labels before purchasing certain food products to limit the risks of eating harmful ingredients.

Good Fats

These are the types of fats that are considered to be healthier to consume. "Good" fats refer to either monounsaturated fats or polyunsaturated fats. When placed at room temperature, these fats tend to stay liquid. A straightforward example of these fats is vegetable oil.

Monounsaturated Fats

Monounsaturated fats are those that contain fewer hydrogen atoms compared to saturated fats. If you look at their chemical structure, they also have a bend at the double bond, as well as a single carbon to carbon double bond. It is these components that make it liquid when the oil is kept at room temperature. Canola, olive, peanut, avocado, high-oleic safflower, and sunflower oils are excellent sources of monounsaturated fats.

The discovery of the health benefits of the monounsaturated oil can be traced back to the Steven Countries Studies of the 1960s when it was discovered that those in Greece and other Mediterranean areas were less susceptible to heart diseases even though their diets were high in fats. The dominant fats in their eating plans were not the saturated animal type that was common in countries with high rates of heart disease; instead, the inhabitants mostly used olive oil, which contained monounsaturated fats. This has made the Mediterranean diet and olive oil the objects of interest to many people and is now considered as healthy options. To replace the effects of saturated and trans fats, experts claim that people should eat as much of monounsaturated fats as possible.

Polyunsaturated Fats

Polyunsaturated fats are regarded as essentials fat because the body needs them to function, although they cannot be produced naturally. Such fats contain two or more double bonds in their carbon chains. They have two types as well: the omega-3 and the omega-6 fatty acids. The unique numbers in these names represent the distance between the beginning of the carbon chain and the first double bond. Polyunsaturated fat is primarily sourced from plant-based foods and oils. It is excellent for heart health as it lowers cholesterol levels and decreases the risk of having cardiovascular disease.

Omega-3 fatty acids have proven to be very beneficial to the heart. Aside from guarding your heart against illnesses, it also lowers the blood pressure and prevents irregular heartbeat. Sardines, salmon, herring, and trout are examples of fish that contain omega-3 fatty acid. If you cannot eat fish, you can also find these polyunsaturated fats in walnuts, flaxseed, and canola oil. Omega-6 fatty acid, on the other hand, is present in roasted soybeans and soy nut butter, walnuts, tofu, margarine, pumpkin seeds, sesame seeds, sunflower seeds, corn oil, sunflower oil, sesame oil, and other vegetable oils.

When polyunsaturated fat is eaten in place of highly refined carbohydrates and saturated fat, the harmful LDL cholesterol levels may decrease, and your cholesterol profile may improve. Also, triglycerides are reduced by this type of good fat. Omega-3 fatty acids may be useful in the treatment of strokes as well. Not only do they raise the HDL level, but they also make sure that your heart rhythm will not dangerously rise. There is evidence that points to the fact that polyunsaturated fats reduce the need for corticosteroid medications of people who suffer from rheumatoid arthritis. There is another research (albeit still inconclusive) that states that omega-3 may improve your chances of avoiding dementia as well (Harvard Health Publishing, 2015).

Chapter 3: Effective Tips for Successful Keto Dieting

You may already know the importance of a keto diet to your health; that's why you are determined to start this therapy. Chances are, you also believe that the journey is going to be a smooth one. Well, even though it is not necessarily challenging to achieve ketosis, it will be foolhardy to think that it is going to be a walk in the park. Since you are entirely new to this path, there is no need to act like an expert, you should be focusing on knowing what to do and how to do it right.

Truth is, the ketogenic diet is not as much about what you do but how well you do it. The better you are at adapting to all the twists and turns of this therapy, the higher the probabilities are of achieving success in a short time. This section takes you through some valuable information on how to reach ketosis and find keto dieting success.

Low Carb Is Everything

The most essential element of the ketogenic diet is the absolute reduction of carbohydrate intake. Though this may not sound super-secret, there are some intricacies that you must learn to execute the process well. While the body relies on glucose or sugar as a fuel source, it can also make use of other reserves like fatty acids and ketones. Glucose is stored in the liver in the form of glycogen and can be converted to energy. When there is a low level of carbs, these glycogen stores are depleted. It lowers the level of insulin in the body, thus forcing a release of fatty acids from fat deposits. The liver then transforms these fatty acids into acetone, acetoacetate, and beta-hydroxybutyrate, which can then be used to fuel some parts of the brain.

For different individuals, there are varying levels of carb restrictions needed to induce ketosis, but the Atkins diet recommends consuming 20 grams of carbs daily or less for about two weeks to induce ketosis. Once you have attained ketosis, you can then add little amounts of carbohydrates to your diet, making sure that you continue to maintain this metabolic process (Spritzler, 2016). A previous study carried out in one week showed that the people who were suffering from type 2 diabetes reduced their carb level to less than 21 grams daily and experienced the excretion of ketones through the urinary glands 27 times more than their baseline levels (Spritzler, 2016). Another study, however, allowed adults with type 2 diabetes to eat 20-50 grams of carbs daily, depending on the number of carbs that kept them in ketosis within a target of 0.5 to 3.0 mmol/L (Spritzler 2016). In contrast to these results, if you are following a keto diet for therapeutic purposes, your carbs should be restricted to less than 5% of calories or 15 grams per day to boost ketone levels. You should try the program under the supervision of a healthcare expert only.

Focus on What's Right

There are a lot of theories in the keto dieting world. For someone who seeks answers and hopes to get the diet right, they may be contradictory. The need to find the correct answers to fitness-related questions should take precedence over everything. You do not want to invest all your energy on practicing what you think is the real keto diet, only to find out later that you are doing something else. You ought to understand the proper process to do the ketogenic program. Thus, you must concentrate on important things (such as the consumption of a high amount of fats) instead of doing rigorous exercises. After researching, you will find that the reason why keto dieters lose weight is that they eat fewer calories than they are used to. No matter what the level of restriction you place on carbs may be, you can merely burn your own fat by depriving yourself of calories. Your focus, therefore, should be on looking for a diet plan that will allow you consume fewer calories without dealing with cravings and feeling hungry - a couple of issues associated to the early stage of the keto diet. Once you manage to find that kind of diet, you already have a sustainable way to lose weight.

To create a caloric-deficit diet, you should consider these two principles:

- Eat satiating foods that are rich in protein and fiber.
- Get rid of all processed foods that are always rich in calories since they are easy to binge on.

One of the reasons why the keto diet promotes weight loss fast is that it follows the ideas mentioned above more than other popular diets. This results in the feeling of being sated in people who are following the keto diet, even though they are consuming fewer calories. They begin to burn excess fat, which is the common end-goal of individuals who are in the program. If you have been on the keto diet for a while, and you are not getting the results that you want, perhaps it is time to focus less on carb restriction and start eating fewer calories than your body requires to maintain your weight. Being in a caloric deficit is one of the essential keys to losing weight while on the keto diet, and the best way to achieve this is by eating keto-friendly foods, which will be discussed below.

Eat Keto-Friendly Foods

As you may already know, keto-friendly meals refer to foods that are extremely low in carbs. This low-carb level varies for each person, but it is typically restricted to 20 grams per day. To maintain this benchmark, however, you will have to tackle your cravings while checking every food that you consume. After all, most of the things you eat contain a lot of carbs. It may be surprising to you to discover that some natural foods you tend to love (like a banana) will drag you closer to and even over the caloric benchmark that has been set. Though they are high calories, and sugar seems to be everywhere, you should not feel discouraged as there are equally delicious meals that can help you stay faithful to your low-carb diet. Here is a list of foods that you ought to think about while following the ketogenic plan:

- Lamb, poultry, eggs, fish, and beef
- Low-carb vegetables, such as spinach, broccoli, kale, and cauliflower
- High-fat dairy products like full-fat cream, hard cheese, butter, and so on
- Avocados, blackberries, raspberries, and

other low-glycemic berries

- Sweeteners like erythritol, monk fruit, and stevia
- High-fat salad dressing, coconut oil, etc.

Some foods that should be avoided because of their high-carb contents are:

- Wheat, rice, cereals, corn, and other grains
- Apples, oranges, bananas, and other fruits
- Maple syrup, honey, agave, and all other types of sugar
- Potatoes, yams, and other tubers

In addition to the keto-friendly foods listed above, there are baked and fried foods that are made from keto flours that originate from coconut, almond, and similar ingredients. Remember that staying away from carbs does not guarantee weight loss. Even when you eat fewer carbohydrates, if you do not maintain a low-caloric level, you may continue to struggle with weight gain. Hence, it is essential to know how much fats, carbs, and proteins you consume daily.

Engage in Physical Activities

Some studies have shown that people on the keto diet also need to engage in a certain level of physical activities for best results. Ketosis, according to these researches, also help in boosting athleticism. When you are more active, you are likely to reach ketosis faster. During exercise, after all, the level of glycogen in the body plummets and are in turn replenished with the level of carbohydrates, which are then converted to glucose before getting transformed into glycogen once more. When there is a low intake of carbs, there is nothing to replace the glycogen that is expended during exercise, so the liver is forced to produce ketones, which are used in place of glycogen to provide fuel for the muscles.

An investigation states that when the ketone concentration in the blood is low, exercise serves as a booster to the level at which ketones are produced. Besides, the ketone levels may rise as well when one works out in a fasted state.

It is important to note, however, that although exercises boost ketones, it may take a while, about four weeks, for the body to fully adjust in making use of ketones and fatty acids as its primary source of fuel. During this period, it may be a good idea to tone down the physical activities intensity temporarily.

Eat More Healthy Fats

To reach ketosis quickly, it is ideal to consume a lot of healthy fats more regularly. Recall that a low-carb keto diet does not rely on the reduction of carbohydrates alone, but also the increase in fat level. When you are on the keto diet, you draw about 65% to 75% of your calories from fats.

The first step to taking an adequate amount of fat is knowing that they are not dangerous. The good fats will not expose you to heart disease or make you gain weight as long as they are not eaten with carbohydrates. As already stated in the previous chapter, though, there are bad fats that should be totally avoided to keep them from endangering your well-being.

Test Your Ketone Levels

It is an absolute fact that people's bodies and metabolisms are different. While some can handle stress better, other individuals cannot. While a few find it difficult to sleep, many people fall to sleep, rest, or relax very quickly. Some are more physically active than others, too.

To ensure that you are correctly following the diet, it is essential to test your ketone levels to establish carbohydrate and protein baselines for your personal tolerance. There are a couple of ways to do this, but the most effective is by using a blood ketone meter. With these apparatuses, you will be able to know your blood ketone level by the pricking a tip of your finger, similar to how a glucometer is used to test blood sugar for diabetics. These devices will establish whether or not you are in nutritional ketosis. You can easily find a *Precision Xtra* or *Keto Mojo*. Both are inexpensive and do not require a prescription to purchase at a pharmacy.

Light nutritional ketosis falls between 0.5-1.5 mmol/L. You'll be getting a decent effect on your weight, but it is not yet at a peak level. Around 1.5 – 3 mmol/L is what's called optimal ketosis and is recommended for maximum weight loss. Within the first two weeks of the strict keto diet, most people find their ketosis level within the range of 0.5-3.0 mmol/L since the body has now been deprived of glucose. It is making use of fat and producing ketones as a byproduct. You should test your blood ketone level once a week, switching between mornings and evenings alternatively, to find out if your system is remaining in ketosis. After your body has fully adopted the keto diet from 4 to 6 weeks, you can now gradually introduce some proteins, sweet potatoes, and even berries to your meal plan. After that, you should test your blood ketone level the following morning to know whether or not you are still in ketosis. If you are, it shows that your body is insensitive to insulin enough to handle extra protein and carbs and always enjoy the benefits that come with being in ketosis. All this information will be beside the point if you don't take the test.

Track Your Macros

People tend to underestimate the number of calories they consume daily. There is always a difference between the calories you think you are getting and the calories that you actually consume. You may feel that you have cut down your caloric intake, but you are still not losing weight. In reality, some people still manage to lose weight on some low-calorie days, even though their subconscious weight-regulating mechanisms manage to get more calories the next day. The result is that you will gain more weight or reach an all-time-high weight loss level that may be difficult to recover from. Sadly, many dieters fail to grasp what is really happening. They start to blame themselves or their diets. The truth is that they only need to take some time and evaluate the amount of food that they are eating to know where adjustments should be made and what food items need to be avoided entirely. You can monitor the things that you eat by employing the use of calorie tracking apps and a scale. By combining both tools, you will be able to devise an accurate knowledge of your food choices and lose weight consistently. This will help you to avoid eating more calories than you might consume if you have measured the food beforehand, and you will also be able to know what your caloric and macronutrient needs are.

When buying a scale, you may want to consider the following features:

1. Make sure it has a conversion button.

Most scales with conversion button usually has the ounce-to-gram or gram-to-ounce conversion button. This will make food measurement easier to follow because most calorie-tracking devices use a mixture of units.

2. Look for an automatic shutoff.

Before buying a scale, make sure to find out if the apparatus has an automatic shutoff feature. If it does, it may be difficult for you to measure food if it switches off on its own. To be on the safe side, look for a device that allows you to either program the automatic shutoff or will enable you to turn it off manually.

3. Choose a scale that has a removable plate.

If you measure wet ingredients, it can be challenging to clean the plate if it is not removable. You will need to wash that part of the scale sometimes to be sure that you don't get sick. It is a good idea to buy a scale with a detachable plate for easy cleaning.

4. Look for the tare function.

It is easier to weigh things on scales that allow you to place plates, bowls, or cups on them.

With the tare function, the scale reverts to zero when you place an item on top of it.

When you take the time to track the weight of the foods you eat, you can ensure that you will be able to meet your weight-loss goals.

Change Your Food Environment

Your food environment is another crucial factor that impacts what and how much you eat. Even with all the necessary mechanisms in place, it is still possible for you to cheat on your diet. It is even easier when you are traveling, or there is a special occasion. This is why it is of utmost importance to be aware of your food environment.

The food environment is:

The physical presence of food that affects a person's diet,

A person's proximity to food store locations,

The distribution of food stores, food service, and any physical entity by which food may be obtained, or

A connected system that allows access to food (Designed for Disease, 2008).

The food environment is also known as the community food environment, nutritional food environment, or local food environment. The retail food environment includes the community level (e.g., presence and locations of food stores, markets, or both) and the consumer level (e.g., healthful, affordable foods in stores, in markets, or in both) (Designed for Disease, 2008). Your food environment is evolving at a faster pace than ever before. The truth is, our brains and bodies are not wired to handle the abundance of food that has become a staple in our modern food environment. There are increasingly extensive options of dishes to choose from: fast foods to processed foods, organic, and gluten-free. They come in all different forms. For someone who is trying to stay faithful to a diet, it's easy to trigger our desires, because they are always readily available, and your brain pushes you to go for foods that do not require you to work for them. If you choose to act on the signals that your mind sends out, you may find yourself going for calorie-dense foods like french fries, pizza, cakes, cookies, etc. This can cause you to snack in between meals to energize yourself and eating more than you should. This often leads to overeating, which results in weight gain. It is as if we keep reminding ourselves that we need to prepare for famine, even though the famine never comes. It's easier to gather calories and gain weight than lose it. You can prevent these surging desires by giving yourself room to stick to the diet to be able to lose weight.

To achieve this, here are some things you may want to consider:

1. Have meal plans

Planning for the foods you will eat at every meal is an excellent way to stay faithful to your keto diet. Whether you are in transit or just at home, you want to prevent yourself from succumbing to food temptations. When you are on vacation, make sure you have premade meals or keto-friendly snacks. If that is not possible, go to restaurants with keto-friendly options. When at home, prepare meal plans (possibly a meal timetable) that give you all the nutrients that you need and nothing more.

2. Keep only keto-friendly foods around

It may be difficult, but sticking with ketogenic foods is not impossible. When hunger sets in, we may be pushed to act against our own will because, at this point, the only thing the body cares about is how to satisfy your cravings. Whatever rules you may have set for yourself rarely matter when you feel hungry. It makes you vulnerable, and it becomes easy to convince yourself to cheat on your diet.

Planning for the worst is the best option in this case. Ensure that keto-friendly foods are the ones that are within your reach. If you are struggling with overeating keto-foods, try to keep the foods that need some level of processing before eating. This way, you will end up eating fewer calories since you may feel discouraged to eat when you know you have to unwrap or prepare a lot of things.

3. Stick to foods you can measure and track

If you think that adding extra oil, cheese, and or meat to your meals does not mean anything, you would be wrong. These extras are also capable of adding to your weight. You should stick to your macronutrient goals by eating what is necessary for you. If you do add anything extra to a meal, track it to keep yourself heading in the right direction.

At first glance, greasy foods may not look as if they pose a threat to your diet. The more you add to each meal, however, the more they add up. These can halt your progression or add on the weight that you have been working so hard to lose.

4. Avoid eating convenient foods impulsively

Since some foods are quite natural to munch on, we seem to keep them close at hand. While they may be suitable for satiating hunger, they are just as dangerous to your diet if you do not learn to control your ingestion rate.

The indulgence of tasty and convenient foods should be kept at a bare minimum. When you know that you have a favorite keto-friendly snack or meal, you must monitor how you eat them. Make sure you do not have more than one serving at your disposal at a particular point in time unless you are planning on having that meal for the next day. For every food that you know that you can eat without stopping, make it difficult for yourself to consume more of it than you can.

5. Chose a meal plan that works for you

It is important to note that there is no one-size-fits-all approach to the keto diet. What has worked for your friend or sibling may not work for you. People are all wired differently, and metabolic processes are as unique as fingerprints. When you are starting your keto journey, take note of those meals that work best for you, and stick with them. You will try various plans before deciding which of them the best fit is for you. While you're at it, try not to be so quick to switch programs. Remember that the first phase of the diet can be a bit delicate, and you don't want to make yourself uncomfortable by using yourself as a lab rat. Once you notice that your system is responding positively to a particular meal plan, keep up with it for as long as possible before moving on to another if you ever feel the need to switch.

A Short message from the Author:

Hey, are you enjoying the book? I'd love to hear your thoughts!

Many readers do not know how hard reviews are to come by, and how much they help an author.

Customer Reviews

★★★★★ 2
5.0 out of 5 stars ▾

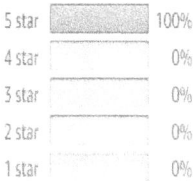

5 star		100%
4 star		0%
3 star		0%
2 star		0%
1 star		0%

See all verified purchase reviews ›

Share your thoughts with other customers

Write a customer review

I would be incredibly thankful if you could take just 60 seconds to write a brief review on Amazon, even if it's just a few sentences!

>> Click here to leave a quick review

Chapter 4: Keto-Friendly Foods

Deciding what to eat when on a keto diet may be tricky as your food choices are now limited to stuff with extremely low carbs. The selection problem aside, without having an idea of what keto-friendly options are available, the whole process may be all for nothing since you may find yourself muddying your diet with foods that you are expected to stay away from in the first place.

We have come up with a list of foods that can be associated with the ketogenic process to help you figure out what to buy and what to eat. While sticking to the 5% carbs rule that comes with the diet, here are the groups of foods you can choose from for your keto-friendly meals.

Proteins

A significant factor to note when it comes to proteins is that the higher the amount of protein in a food, the lesser the quantity of that food consumed should be. When you limit your protein intake to pasture-raised and grass-fed options, you minimize the risk of taking in bacteria and steroid hormones that other meat products have. In red meats, there isn't too much to be scared of. Although added sugar, salt, and other processed ingredients are found in cured meats. When buying steaks, consider going for fatter cuts like the rib-eye. Ground beef for hamburgers or other meals, fattier ratios like 85:15 or 80:20 are advised. For poultry, darker meats contain more fat than white varieties, so it is better to stick to them. Whitefishes, on the other hand, are not only rich in protein but also give you Omega-3.

Remember that you do not need too much protein when you are on a keto diet as they lead to lower levels of ketones and an increased level of glucose. With this in mind, when dealing with meat, make sure you are mindful of protein intake. Keep in mind that you are aiming for nutritional ketosis. You can, however, play an easy trick by trying to balance out your proteins and eating fattier side dishes. If you decide to eat lean beef, you will have to be careful with the proportion of protein. Do not forget that jerky and other beef snacks can pile up your protein level fast as well, so make sure to accompany it with a portion of fatty food like cheese.

If you do not eat pork or beef, lamb can be substituted in its place. Cuts of meat like bacon can be replaced with similar leaner items, too. You can add extra fat if you deem it necessary.

To get protein on a ketogenic diet, here are some options to look into:

- Beef: Use steaks with fattier cuts wherever possible. Roasts, ground beef, stew meats, and steaks are good ideas.
- Poultry: Duck, pheasant, quail, chicken, and any other wild game.
- Fish: Anything caught in the wild like catfish, halibut, mackerel, flounder, mahi-mahi, cod, trout, snapper, tuna, and salmon.
- Shellfish: Oysters, crabs, lobsters, scallops, mussels, squid, and clams.
- Pork: When consuming pork, be on the lookout for added sugars and stick to the fattier cuts. Pork chops, ground pork, ham, pork loin, and tenderloins are a wonderful source of protein.
- Offal/organs: These are very excellent sources of vitamins and other nutrients. They are made up of the internal organs of an animal, including heart, kidney, liver, and tongue.

- Bacon and sausage: Check the labels and watch out for anything cured in sugar or those that have other fillers.
- Whole eggs: If possible, get free range from the local market. There is a variety of ways to prepare them, such as scrambled, poached, fried, boiled, and deviled.
- Nut butter: It is better to go for natural and unsweetened while sticking with the fattier options like almond butter and macadamia butter. Be careful with the consumption of legumes (e.g., peanuts) as they are high in omega-6.
- Other Meats: You should stick to fattier cuts of turkey, veal, lamb, goat, and other wild game.

When you do eat meat, it is fine to have it in moderation. Always remember that the intake of proteins must be in balance with fat.

Fats and Oils

Recall what we have already discussed about good and bad fats in the second chapter. When choosing your foods, it is essential to apply your knowledge regarding their differences by choosing to obtain fats from natural sources like fruits and nuts. You can also use ingredients like butter, coconut oil, olive oil, etc.

When on a ketogenic diet, fats and oils will be the majority of your daily caloric intake. It is crucial to keep the things you like or dislike under consideration while creating your meals. There are several ways to add fats and oils to your meals, either in the form of toppings or dressings. For polyunsaturated and monounsaturated fats, to be specific, foods like egg yolk, coconut oil, olive oil, macadamia, avocado, and nuts are less inflammatory and chemically stable for most people.

It's important to balance your consumption of omega-3 and omega-6 as well; that's why you should go for fish such as tuna, trout, wild salmon, and shellfish. If you are not a fan of seafood (or you are allergic to them), you may choose to take fish oil supplements. Krill oil is also a good source of omega-3. Fruits and nuts, however, can be extremely high in omega-6 so you may want to eat sources like peanuts, pine nuts, walnuts, and almonds in moderation. Safflower and corn oils are also excellent sources of omega-6 as well. To keep your fatty acids at a healthy range, you should not overindulge in desserts that have a high concentration of almond flour. Even though these essential fatty acids provide humans with some core nutrients, they are mostly not balanced in a standard diet.

Here are some fresh ideas for keto-friendly foods that are rich in good fats and oils:

- Coconut butter
- Olive oil
- Cocoa butter
- MCT
- Avocado oil
- Macadamia oil
- Coconut oil
- Olive oil
- Macadamia/Brazil nuts
- Mayonnaise
- Butter/Ghee
- Egg yolks
- Tallow
- Fatty fish
- Avocado
- Lard
- Animal fat (non-hydrogenated)

When you are making use of vegetable oils that come from soybeans, safflower, flax or olive, it is better to go for "cold-pressed" options if they are available. In case you prefer to fry things up, you should choose non-hydrogenated lard, ghee, coconut oil, or beef tallow since these oils have higher smoke points than other types. A higher smoke point means that you will get a greater concentration of essential fatty acids from them.

Fruits and Vegetables

Vegetables are a crucial part of the keto diet, but there are times when we get stuck because of some decisions made and regret them later. Green, leafy vegetables remain the best option when it comes to selecting the right sources for your keto-friendly meals. Some vegetables are very high in sugar and do not contribute positively to our diet, so the decision to cut those out of your diet is vital for the program's success. When following a ketogenic diet, eating vegetables that are high in nutrients and low in carbohydrates are the best options. These can be included in almost every meal as well. They are mostly leafy and dark vegetables - anything that shares semblance with spinach or kale. It is a good idea to go for cruciferous vegetables that are grown above the ground.

Organically grown vegetables are good, as they do not have pesticide residue. Besides the harmful chemicals, though, there is not much difference between the organic and non-organic varieties. As research has shown, their nutritional qualities are the same. This means that there is no need to feel too bothered if you cannot get the organically grown vegetables as the non-organic ones are just as good. Both frozen and fresh options are available year round, so there are not many limitations when it comes to choosing what to eat. If you wish to consume vegetables that have grown below the ground, you should do so in moderation. To be specific, you need to be careful with the number of carbohydrates that they have. Often, underground vegetables are used as flavorings for foods and are very easy to regulate. For example, you can use half an onion for a whole pot of soup.

When choosing your vegetables, you should divvy up your choices according to their carb rate. You should try as much as you can to limit your intake of the following fruits and vegetables:

- High-carb vegetables: garlic, onion, mushroom, parsnip, potatoes, starchy vegetables, and squash
- Citrus: orange, lemon, and lime in both

juice and recipes
- Nightshades: eggplant, pepper, and tomatoes
- Fruits: bananas, blackberries, raspberries, strawberries, and blueberries

Some of the most common keto-friendly vegetables are cabbage, cauliflower, broccoli, romaine lettuce, spinach, baby bella mushrooms, green bell pepper, yellow onions, and green beans.

Dairy Products

Milk-based products are mostly keto-friendly, so any type is acceptable. You may, however, want to stick to full-fat dairy items.

Dairy products are consumed with other meals on the keto diet as they are not to be eaten as main dishes, but you should consume them at a minimal level. Typically, most of the meals in this plan come from fats/cooking oils, proteins, and vegetables. When eating dairy products, it is preferable to eat organic choices since the processed ones always have about two to five times higher levels of carbohydrates, and they add up with time. Full-fat dairy products are preferable as opposed to low fat or fat-free products, which have significantly higher levels of carbohydrates. If you are sensitive to lactose, it is better to go for long-aged dairy products because they have less lactose concentration. Examples of dairy items that can be eaten when following a keto diet are:

- Hard cheeses: aged cheddar, parmesan, Swiss, feta, and so on
- Soft cheeses: Brie, Colby, Monterey Jack, blue, and mozzarella
- Spreadable: cream cheese, mascarpone, crème Fraiche, sour cream, etc.
- Heavy whipping cream
- Mayonnaise and mayo alternatives that are also rich in dairy
- Greek yogurt

If you are looking for ways to add extra fat to your meal, you can prepare fatty side dishes or sauces like creamed spinach. Keep in mind; however, they are rich in protein as well, so you have to be careful when pairing them with foods that are already loaded with protein.

It is essential to pay close attention to your body when consuming dairy products. If you have noticed that you have either reached a plateau or slowed down in losing weight, you may have to think about reducing your dairy intake.

Nuts and Seeds

First of all, you should know that peanuts are prohibited in the keto diet because they are legumes. That said, nuts are best consumed when roasted since the process removes harmful nutrients and reduces their level of acidity. Raw nuts are mostly used as flavorings to foods and for adding texture. You can have them for snacks as well. While this may be rewarding, it may be a bad idea for your weight-loss goal since nuts may work against it in the long run. Snacking on nuts generally raises the level of insulin in your body. That's why they may slow down your ability to lose extra pounds. While they are a great source of fats, it is vital to keep in mind that they also have carbohydrates and proteins. Protein in nut flours, in particular, can quickly accumulate; when using them, you have to be aware of the amount that you use. Omega-6 fatty acids are also one of the nutrients found in nuts. Typically, you may want to consider sticking with the fattier options since they happen to have a lower amount of carbohydrates.

Here are things to consider before deciding to open a bag of nuts when you are on a ketogenic diet:

- Brazil nuts, macadamia nuts, and pecans are fatty, low-carb choices. They can be eaten with meals or as fat supplements.
- Hazelnuts, pine nuts, and walnuts contain a moderate amount of carbohydrates. They should be eaten only for texture or flavor.

- Cashews and pistachios are to be avoided or rarely eaten as they have a very high concentration of carbohydrates. Cashews, for instance, has almost as many carbs as you need to survive for an entire day.

Brazil nuts, pecans, macadamia nuts, almonds, and hazelnuts are the most common keto friendly nuts available.

Nuts and seed flours are excellent substitutes for regular flours. In keto, seeds and nuts are often associated with baked desserts. Almond flours and flaxseed meals are standard products used, but it's essential to eat them at a moderate level. You can experiment with your baking recipes by mixing different flours to get a consistent texture that will mimic wheat flour. This mixture will lead to lower carb counts in recipes. You should be aware of the fact that flours react differently. Primarily when used in baking. While coconut flour, for instance, will absorb more water, almond flour will not require as much liquid. These flours are not only useful for baking alone, but you can use them to coat your meat before frying. Also, they can serve as the base for foods like pizza. With enough creativity, you will be able to recreate an old-time favorite by creating a low carb version of it.

Almond flour, coconut flour, chia seed meal, flaxseed meal, unsweetened coconut, etc. are some of the keto-friendly nut/seed items you may consider choosing from.

Water and Other Beverages

For beverages, water is always the best idea. Not only does it keep you healthier, but it is more hydrating than anything else. You may decide to add flavorings to your water by adding lime/lemon juice.

For most people who have started trying the ketogenic diet, dehydration is a widespread side effect that's caused by the natural diuretic effect of the program. If you are prone to bladder pain and urinary tract infections, you are advised to prepare more for this if you wish to go on the keto diet. For the first weeks, prepare yourself to drink at least eight glasses of water daily. This is very important to stay hydrated, so you should drink more water than you are probably used to while following the ketogenic process.

If you can recall, dehydration and the lack of electrolytes are significant causes of keto flu. Considering two-thirds of the human body is made up of water, experts advise that people should stay hydrated all day, regardless of whether you are on the keto diet or not. It depends on your size, weight, activity level, and where you live. In general, you should try to drink between half an ounce and an ounce of water for each pound you weigh, every day. For example, if you weigh 150 pounds, that would be 75 to 150 ounces of water a day. If you live in a hot climate and exercising a lot, you'd be on the higher end of that range; if you're in a colder climate and mostly sedentary, you'd need less. (Nessler, 2009). For many individuals, keto approved beverages and coffee do the trick to up their energy rate and added fats. To help stay hydrated, replace one serving of a caffeinated drink with a glass of water. You will also need to be conscious of the fact that you need to replenish your electrolytes by drinking bone broth or sports drinks that are flavored with sucralose or stevia.

Below are some examples of keto-friendly beverages:

- Water: This is your everyday source of hydration. As one of the building blocks of life, it is easily accessible to you. You may choose to drink either sparkling or regular water.
- Bone broth: This liquid provides electrolytes that can kick start your energy. It is also loaded with nutrients and vitamins.
- Coffee: With some added weight loss benefits, this beverage helps in improving your mental focus.
- Tea: Even though not many people find this enjoyable, it has the same effects as coffee. If you choose to drink tea, try to stick with white or green tea. It has less caffeine than other teas do as well as added weight loss and health benefits.

- Coconut/Almond Milk: This can easily replace your favorite beverage. The unsweetened versions are your best options.
- Flavorings: Those packets that are flavored with sucralose or stevia are the best when it comes to taste. Alternatively, you may add a squeeze of orange, lime, or lemon to your water bottle.
- Alcohol: Try to stay away from beer and wine as much as you can. If you must drink alcohol, go for hard liquor. Nonetheless, remember that too much alcohol will slow down your weight-loss process.

Spices, Seasonings, and Condiments

Spices and seasonings are a fundamental part of everyday cooking. Without them, food would be bland and unenjoyable. Who wants to eat plain chicken? When it comes to the keto diet, though, it can be very tricky. Even though they may come off as small ingredients, they are capable of adding extra carbs to a meal. If you wish to be strict with your seasonings, ultimately you will have to consider staying away from processed foods. Even though there seems to be a lot of low-carb condiments in the market, most of them have a high concentration of glycemic sweeteners, and you may want to avoid them.

When you are tracking your overall carb level, you should add spices to your calculations because they also contain carbohydrates. Often, premade spice mixtures contain sugars, so be sure to go through the nutrition label before consuming them to know what they are. For salt, you can choose sea salts over table salts as they are often powdered with dextrose. If you can, do not add more sugar to your spice blend or foods.

Below are some common keto-friendly spices and seasonings.

- Rosemary
- Oregano
- Cayenne pepper
- Cinnamon
- Cumin
- Basil
- Chili powder
- Parsley
- Thyme

- Cilantro

Consequently, you can add salt and pepper to your food without much worries about their nutritional information.

It will always be better for you on a keto diet to stick to homemade foods than processed ones. The more real food you consume, the more you can control the ingredients that go in it. Even though it is acceptable to consume processed foods, many of them out there are not very good for the keto diet. For this reason, you should check food labels before buying or consuming anything.

Chapter 5: Keto Friendly Meals

If you have come this far with us, then it's safe to say that you are prepared to go head-on into the ketogenic program. The success of your journey largely depends on the food that you eat, as well as the proportions and nutritional values of the foods that you consume. To help you, we have combined a list of keto friendly meals, broken down into breakfast, lunch, and dinner ideas. You will find an extensive variety of food in this section, and most of them should be easily accessible to you.

Breakfast

Before setting out to make your ketogenic breakfast, you should ask yourself: do you want your food to get prepared with minimal cooking or not cooked at all? You can make meals that you can finish up in five minutes, and the good thing is that breakfasts generally cook quickly, so it is a win-win situation. Below are some breakfast ideas that may work for you.

Eggs

The only nutrient that will be missing in your egg meal is a vitamin. It pretty much has all the nutrients that you need, and you can make it by boiling, scrambling, or frying. For a healthy, highly satiating meal, you can choose to add some leafy vegetables as well. You should consider adding other fat sources, such as butter, mayonnaise, or olive oil, to feel full for hours.

If you choose to have breakfast without eggs, there are several other options available for you. You can also try raw nuts, avocados, olives, cheese, smoked salmon, or mackerel. All of these are examples of nutrient-laden meals that you can try, and they are bound to keep you satisfied until lunchtime.

Breakfast Pizza

You do not need pepperoni or cheese to make a keto-friendly pizza. It is a perfect breakfast recipe that uses a cauliflower base and is loaded with avocado, smoked salmon, and runny eggs. With this meal, you can get as much as 7 grams of carbs, together with other nutrients, which makes it a balanced breakfast with coffee or tea.

Collagen Bread

After enjoying this zero-carb bread, you will believe in the existence of miracles. You can either smother it in butter or low-carb strawberry jam or use it as a base for breakfast sandwiches with avocado, fish, bacon or eggs.

Cauliflower Bread with Crispy Bacon, Avocado, and Poached Eggs

Even though most keto cauliflower bread uses shredded cheese or heavy cream to bind them together, this one is 100% dairy-free. Using a little bit of cauliflower rice and psyllium husk, you can create a hash brown-style base for runny eggs and crispy bacon. It contains about 5.5 grams of net carbs.

Rosemary Bagel

This is another excellent food that is best served after smearing grass-fed butter or stacking meat and eggs on top. The spongy texture of herby bagels comes from a combination of almond flour, xanthan gum, and psyllium husk. The great part is that you can enjoy this keto breakfast recipe at only 9 grams of net carbs per bagel.

Cinnamon Sugar Doughnuts with Almond Flour

These cake-like doughnuts have the perfect crumb and light crunch from a dusting of cinnamon sugar. Having only 3 grams of net carbs per doughnut, you can sneak in an extra one to dunk in your coffee without feeling guilty. You can swap coconut milk for almond milk, as well as utilize grass-fed butter and non-GMO erythritol to make the recipe keto friendly.

Keto Chocolate Doughnuts

Although tender, chocolate-filled doughnuts are perfect on their own, this breakfast recipe gets enhanced with a rich, sweet glaze. You can enjoy them when combined with coffee and tea or eaten as a dessert. With a little over 2 grams of carbs per doughnut, it will not affect your progress if you want to indulge. If you wish to try other varieties, you can make use of grass-fed butter and coffee or change heavy cream with full-fat coconut milk for the glaze.

Classic Bulletproof/Butter Coffee

Bulletproof or butter coffee is an incredible way to begin your day. This recipe is so magical that it causes us to get up in the morning. We have learned not only the official recipe for bulletproof coffee but also the reasons why it works to suppress hunger and how it switches on the brain. It is absolutely carb-free.

Adaptogenic Bulletproof/Butter Coffee

This is a spin on the original bulletproof coffee, which makes use of adaptogens to lift up your mood and help you fight fatigue. Also, the beverage has anti-inflammatory turmeric and vanilla bean that can make the start of your day both sweet and satisfying. This keto breakfast contains about a gram of carbs.

Bulletproof/Butter Coffee Egg Latte

You probably have the urge to exclaim, "Raw eggs? In coffee?" Well, you will never get to find out how tasty this combo is if you do not give it a try. With egg yolk, you get a satisfying creaminess, after all, while healthy fat is added to this keto breakfast recipe. It may also pass as a post-workout drink, considering you consume a gram of carb per mug.

Iced Macha Latte

Despite its cool and creamy nature, an iced matcha latte still delivers a dose of caffeine while supplying healthy fats from coconut milk. Each mug gives about 4.8 grams of net carbs and is an excellent pair for a full plate of bacon.

Anti-Inflammatory Spiced Chai Latte

With earthy turmeric, this recipe contains a golden hue, as well as fuel from fat. It also has gut-healing benefits from gelatin and collagen and is a caffeine-free alternative that's easy on the stomach. It only contains about 3 grams of total carbs.

CBD Rooibos Tea Latte

Cannabidiol (CBD) oil is an optional breakfast recipe, but including it to your diet can be a perfect way to start the day. Caffeine-free rooibos tea gets upgraded with grass-fed ghee, collagen, and CBD oil to create a warm and creamy latte, which is capable of helping you to keep your cool. The best part of it is that it only has a gram of carb per serving.

Fluffy Almond Flour Pancakes

With notes of vanilla and cinnamon, this is a keto breakfast recipe that the entire family can enjoy. Also, it is easy to combine the ingredients. You will first have to blend all the items together and then spoon the batter onto a greased griddle pan. This meal provides about 4.5 grams of net carbs for each serving, and it is the best solution for your pancake cravings.

Coconut Flour Crepes

These light and thin crepes are perfect options to be used as a base for low-sugar berries or coconut whipped cream. To make this breakfast more keto-friendly, you can use water or coconut milk instead of almond milk. This recipe also gives you about a gram of carb per crepe.

Strawberry-Chocolate Crepes

Light and sweet crepes get star treatment from a thick, dark chocolate sauce and chunks of fresh strawberries. Best of all, this indulgent recipe only provides 5 grams of net carbs. Use grass-fed butter (or dairy-free coconut oil) to keep this breakfast bulletproof.

Paleo Chocolate Almond Butter Crepes

Are you running short of berries? There's no need to worry since this keto breakfast has your crepes swimming in a thick almond butter-based chocolate sauce. This meal provides approximately 3 grams of net carbs per filled crepe, and the recipe is straightforward and keto-friendly. Make use of full-fat coconut milk, raw almond butter, or grass-fed butter to make it Bulletproof.

Buttery Coconut Flour Waffles

Mixing coconut flour, non-dairy milk, and eggs can turn into crisp and fluffy waffles. With about 4 grams of net carbs in each waffle, this keto meal makes the perfect addition to a plate of bacon and eggs. To give a bulletproof spin on this recipe, you can make use of full-fat coconut milk and grass-fed butter as your dairy choices

Bacon-and-Egg Fat Bombs

Fat bombs don't need to be too sweet. This savory keto breakfast recipe uses something like an egg salad mixture and surrounds it with bits of crisp bacon for a fun take on the original bacon-and-eggs variety. It contains 2 grams of net carbs and is absolutely keto-friendly. You can make use an avocado oil-based mayo to keep these little bites bulletproof.

Bacon-and-Egg Breakfast Muffins

Egg muffins are the perfect make-ahead keto breakfast to keep you on track. Plus, they're easy to customize. With only 4 grams of net carbs per cup, you can enjoy it either in the morning or during nighttime. You only need to ensure that you use pastured bacon to make it healthier.

Bacon Hash

You can turn chopped cauliflower into a savory potato alternative in this take on a breakfast hash. It only requires 15 minutes to prepare, and it serves as a brilliant option for weekday mornings or weekend brunches. If you wish to make this keto breakfast recipe bulletproof, you only need to use pastured bacon.

Keto Breakfast Wrap

This recipe uses a combination of a layer of egg omelet and avocado in a neat nori sheet so that you can have a breakfast on-the-go. Although the avocado and nori add filling fiber to the meal, the entire meal merely contains 2 grams of net carbs.

Egg Crepes with Avocados

This meal takes a flour-free approach to crepes by using a cooked egg to wrap up layers of mayo, meat, and avocado. You only obtain a gram of carb from one whole crepe. If you are considering to keep it bulletproof, make use of pastured bacon instead of turkey, and then add avocado oil mayo. Cook your egg gently, too.

Lemon Blueberry Muffins

This moist and hearty vanilla cake gets studded with fresh and sweet blueberries. What else can you look for in a keto breakfast recipe? With about 6 grams of carbs per muffin, these glazed bites can become the highlight of your morning.

Dairy-Free Keto Chocolate Muffins

These little cakes stay moist with fiber-filled pumpkin, which turns them into a delicious keto breakfast that is capable of silencing your chocolate cravings. It has added collagen peptides that can smooth your skin and strengthen your hair and nails. You can enjoy all these benefits by merely consuming 3 grams of carbs per muffin.

Crisp Cinnamon Toast Crunch Cereal

You should be excited to see that low-carb cereals have finally arrived. This keto breakfast idea is lovely and munchable, all thanks to a crispy dough that is made from almond flour, warm cinnamon, and grass-fed butter. It contains 2 grams of carbs per serving only and is a significant upgrade from the boxed stuff, taste and nutrition-wise.

Chocolate-Coconut Keto Smoothie Bowl

This is a creamy, dreamy keto breakfast recipe that tastes like dessert and fills your bowl with healthy fat and protein from coconut milk and collagen peptides. It only contains 8 grams of net carbs. Eating this meal will make you feel as good as it looks.

Keto Green Smoothie

Begin your day with a whopping 6 grams of fiber and 8 grams of carbs from a keto green smoothie. This liquid meal combines frozen avocado chunks and a spicy ginger blend together with green veggies for a filling, frosty breakfast substitute. If you desire to stay bulletproof, make use of organic spinach and steam it lightly before adding to your blender.

Low-Carb Cucumber Green Tea Detox Smoothie

This comes with a caffeinated touch from matcha powder and creaminess from the avocado. It is an emerald-colored keto breakfast recipe that is perfect for any morning and not just for detoxification purposes. Make use of high-quality matcha without sweeteners to keep this smoothie bulletproof.

Lunch

Unlike breakfasts, lunchtime meals are not usually as light, and they often require more effort to put together. In this section, we will give you some details about keto-friendly lunch recipes that will make it easier to commit to your health goals than ever.

Loaded Chicken Salad

From golden-brown chicken and lightly grilled asparagus, down to the fresh avocado chunks and creamy spheres of mozzarclla, this protcin-laden meal is the best keto lunch idea. With every bite, you are bound to get an explosion of flavors in your mouth and always look forward to munching on every last bit of the salad during mealtime.

Zucchini Crust Grilled Cheese

Thanks to the carb-free bread slices that can be made with mozzarella, parmesan, and grated cheddar sitting right in the middle, grilled cheese isn't here to mess around. There is no need to worry about balance because, in each sandwich, you have two cups of grated zucchini as a part of the bread. Therefore, you can get an ample amount of vegetables along with the cheeses.

Salad with Roasted Cauliflower

It may be quite tasking to be on a keto diet and stay vegan at the same time, but with recipes like the salad with roasted cauliflower, it is not an impossible thing to do. With lots of olive oil, nuts, and avocado to provide those satisfying, healthy fats, the cauliflower becomes better and more pleasing to munch on than leafy greens.

Shrimp Avocado Salad

It takes only 15 minutes to prepare this meal and, within that short period, only five minutes is spent on actual cooking. Once the shrimp is stirred in the butter, you only need to dice the vegetables and make the dressing. It's super easy, fast, and filled with the best flavors.

Keto Chicken Enchilada Bowl

If you are going on a keto diet, make up your mind to become friends with cauliflower. It is the ingredient that makes these meals possible. In place of rice, and topped with some saucedup chicken, avocado, and cheese, it allows you to stay carb-free while still enjoying an enchilada.

Keto Quesadillas

These are almost exactly like regular tortillas, but the wraps for these cheesy wedges are actually made from mostly eggs and coconut flour. Once the quesadillas win your heart over, feel free to use the tortilla for other dishes like soft tacos.

Sesame Salmon with Baby Bok Choy and Mushrooms

You may need 30 minutes to prepare this meal, but it gets to serve you for as long as the next four lunchtimes, so this is an absolutely time-saving recipe. The longer you let the salmon and vegetables sit in the marinade, the tastier they will become with every day that passes. Be sure that you can use up all the fish by the fourth day to prevent it from going in the trash.

Salmon and Avocado Nori Rolls

Are you used to including sushi on your meals every week before you have decided to go on the keto diet? If your answer is yes, you do not have much to miss out on. You can make keto-friendly rolls, too. All you need to do is to exclude rice from your roll, and then allow the salmon, avocado, and cucumber to play the lead roles.

Caprese Tuna Salad Stuffed Tomatoes

Coated in balsamic vinegar instead of mayo, this Italian-inspired tuna salad is a very viable option for you when you want to take your lunch to work. Stuffed in tomatoes, it's not just a perfect low-carb option. It also scores some points when it comes to the presentation as the colors are appealing to the eyes.

Caprese Eggplant Panini with Lemon Basil Aioli

With your new keto lifestyle, you can increase your vegetable intake in some very creative ways. In this recipe, to be specific, the egg is replaced with eggplant, while the classic Panini goodies like mozzarella, basil, and tomato are tucked inside. You can serve it with creamy garlic aioli. Voila, your gourmet lunch is ready.

Cinnamon Pork Chops and Mock Apples

You may have presumed that pork chops and apples are more suitable for dinner, but that is not entirely true. This meal idea shows how it can be made to become a perfect option even for lunch. Before you object that apples aren't keto-friendly, note that you can use the chayote squash with cinnamon and nutmeg instead of the real fruit.

Spicy Kimchi Ahi Poke

Because your body's still adjusting to the high-fat lifestyle, your digestion may require a bit of nudge. To help it along, you should keep your gut health in check with probiotic-rich foods like kimchi. This fermented cabbage can do wonders for your stomach. When it is mixed with a bit of mayo, tuna, and avocado, it passes for a pretty awesome lunch.

Spinach Mozzarella Stuffed Burgers

Do you want to know how it can be possible for you to contain your cheeseburger fixings without the bread? It's easy. The best advice is to take the Juicy Lucy route. You just need to stuff the greens and the cheese inside the beef patty, instead of piling it on top. Not only does it give you a great taste, but it also makes eating more fun this way.

Low-Carb Mexican Meatza

The traditional pizza might be off-limits for you on the keto diet, but since life without pizza doesn't seem to ever be an option, here's an excellent alternative for you: the low-carb Mexican meatza. The crust is made with cauliflower and has ground beef to give you some protein. Your fat sources in this recipe are the avocado and cheddar toppings, which can supply your ketogenic needs.

Easy Keto Egg Salad

Because the focus of the keto diet is on high-fat and moderate-protein meals, a ketogenic dieter needs a good egg salad recipe up their sleeve. This one is just perfect since it makes use of avocado for extra heart-healthy fatty acids, as well as dill for a boost of fresh flavor.

Low-Carb Chicken Philly Cheesesteak

Do away with the bread and load up on the filling, which is the best part of this chicken Philly cheesesteak-in-a-bowl anyway. With this meal, you have everything you need, from the meat and the Worcestershire sauce to the provolone and the peppers, so you don't ever have to miss the hoagie roll.

Easy Asiago Cauliflower Rice

There are three keywords in this recipe. Cheese. Cream. Rice. Well, this is not precisely rice but riced cauliflower, so once you cook it and coat it with the said cheese and cream, we can guarantee that you'd never be able to tell the difference.

Keto Broccoli Soup with Turmeric and Ginger

Get a thermos and fill it with this creamy, six-ingredient broccoli soup. Thanks to the coconut milk, you will surely leave your taste buds dancing for joy, and the anti-inflammatory turmeric and ginger will make your immune system happy too.

Keto Chili

This make-ahead, slow-cooker chili makes up for the beans that are lacking in your diet. Adding ground sausage with the ground beef makes for a really meaty meal. Just make sure that your tomato paste doesn't have any added sugars because they are absolutely not allowed on the keto diet.

Dinner

After a long day at work, you obviously do not want to come home to a boring meal. Dinners are your last chance to fill up before your day ends. Here are some great ideas to be sure that all your effort throughout the rest of the day is not wasted.

Sesame Chicken

Everyone who is a fan of Chinese food will have some idea of what sesame chicken is, as well as how good it tastes. The problem is that the regular variety will most likely have more carbohydrates in it. To make it keto-friendly, you can have the breaded sesame chicken with a large portion of veggies.

Creamy Chicken Bacon Casserole

If you are a lover of chicken and bacon, imagine how good they will be if you eat them together in a casserole. You can go through this meal for days on end without concern. Note that without some kind of vegetables mixed into it, it will not be a casserole. For this recipe, you will need a pound of broccoli. The latter may prevent the dish from lasting for too long, but there is nothing wrong with devouring leftovers, especially if they taste this good.

Oven-Baked Chicken Avocado Casserole

The good thing about casseroles is that almost no varieties are the same. There are so many combinations of foods that you can combine into one. You can choose to add anything together, throw it in the oven, add some cheese on top, and voila, your casserole is ready. Casseroles are unique because they can have superfoods in them, including avocados, which are one of the healthiest foods on the planet. It's filled with numerous vitamins and minerals that are significant contributors to your overall health. If you like guacamole, then you'll love the taste of a chicken avocado casserole.

Bacon Cheeseburger Casserole

Consider this recipe as something similar to a burger pie. It is going to be slightly time-consuming to make, but it will last you for days, so it is worth your time and effort. If you think you have to eat a lot to keep up with your macros, you'll still have plenty of leftovers to go through, so don't worry about that. In each bite, you will get the taste of a cheeseburger without the bun.

Chicken Cordon Bleu

Consider getting a little fancy by making an oven-baked chicken cordon bleu. If you've never had it in the past, you should know that it comes with a fantastic combination of chicken and ham. Yes, you guessed right: it tastes just as good as it sounds! When the juices from both types of meat mix together, they make for one of the most delicious meals you will ever eat so there will be no surprise when it becomes one of your favorites.

Stuffed Pork Chops

Pork chops are great, but they can get a little boring sometimes if you continue to eat the same type all the time. For this reason, you may consider switching it up a bit. Pork chops are all-time-favorite meals, but what do you think about stuffing them? You have to ensure that you cook the pork all the way through since you cannot prepare a stuffed version in the same way that you make a typical pork chop. That's the way things are, but once you have cooked the pork chops correctly, you will feel fulfilled, knowing that you have prepared a fantastic meal.

Parmesan-Dijon Crusted Pork Chops

When you're able to get an effective breading on your protein aside from breadcrumbs, you will have to take advantage of this recipe. Adding breading to anything is going to give a bit of crunch that may be missing in other recipes. You will, therefore, be happily surprised with how your recipe turns out.

Keto Lime Pork Chops

Although you might initially think that the lime flavor doesn't go well with pork chops, you should not knock the idea out until you try it. You'll discover that the combination works surprisingly well.

Creamy Mustard Lemon Pork

If you want a slice of tender pork that is filled with flavor, cooking creamy mustard lemon pork is always a great idea. Perfecting this recipe will give you a tender piece of meat that will gently melt in your mouth with every bite you take. Try not to drool over yourself when the recipe turns out well.

Cumin-Spiced Beef Wraps

These beef wraps can act as either a full meal or a quick snack, depending on the amount you choose to make. Though the recipe comes in 8 wraps, it counts for just 2 servings. The wraps themselves will be lettuce, which is perfect for this keto diet. It may not have the same consistency as a regular tortilla or something similar, but the taste is going to come out almost the same. Lettuce wraps replace flour tortillas, and there will be no regretting it.

Cheeseburger Calzone

If you love calzones and/or cheeseburgers, then you will need to try this recipe. A big, meaty calzone that tastes like a cheeseburger is something that some people may consider a dream, but this recipe proves that it can happen. One of the best parts about this cheeseburger calzone is that, when made correctly, you can get up to 8 servings. This meal can last you for one week or a few days, depending on how often you munch on it.

Swedish Meatballs

Who doesn't love to have a good meatball from time to time? Even if you don't like meatballs, give this recipe a try because it tastes that good and you deserve to have it. Meatballs will go with almost anything, and this Swedish recipe is perfect for you.

Stuffed and Wrapped Shrimp

Shrimp is one of our favorite keto-friendly meals. When great flavors are added to an already delicious entree, your taste buds may pop up gleefully to thank you. This recipe for jalapeno stuffed shrimp wrapped in bacon is easy to follow. Since the bacon doesn't take too long to cook, you can have a delicious meal waiting for you in a few minutes.

Shrimp Scampi

When starting with the keto diet, you need to tap into the recipes that remind you of the menu that you used to be on before starting the new one. We are specifically talking about dishes that will remind you of carbohydrates, such as shrimp scampi. Using zucchini, though, you will make a meal of noodles, which looks similar to regular noodles. This way, it may feel like you are eating the real version of the dish.

Salmon Curry

Did you know that you can make an excellent curry dish with seafood? The salmon curry is absolutely a must-try for those who enjoy curry. You can easily replace the rice with riced cauliflower or other riced veggies.

Seafood Soup

Generally, seafood is great for the keto diet. Nevertheless, it is going to taste even better when put in soup, regardless of the broth used. Since it incorporates both seafood and broth, you probably won't mind sipping it all day.

Chapter 6: Intermittent Fasting

Intermittent fasting has become a new craze in the world of fitness. According to theories, it helps people to stay fit, live longer, and even lose weight. Unlike the ketogenic diet, intermittent fasting is not a diet plan since it does not provide restrictions to what you eat. It practically focuses on a modern approach to eating and fasting. There are many health benefits to this dietary plan, including weight loss. However, before starting it, you should find out if it is suitable for you since it is not always a healthy choice for everybody. In summary, intermittent fasting, unlike other weight-loss therapies, is a pattern that circles around the way you eat, regardless of your food choices.

Although there is no standard duration for fasting, the most common intermittent fasts involve fasting for 16 hours every day or 24 hours two times a week. Whenever you find yourself not eating, you are fasting. This can take place between breakfast and lunch or lunch and dinner. Naturally, humans are wired to be able to function for long hours without food. In fact, history proves that ancient hunters could carry on for days in the wild without food, as they couldn't preserve it for consumption later. This made them have to fast until they could get something to eat again. Fasting for religious purposes is also seen in modern society. Fasting is seen as a more natural phenomenon than that of the practice of eating three to four times daily and can be taken as a part of everyday life.

There is a need to distinguish fasting from starvation since some people may think that they are the same thing. Fasting is a controlled absence of food for a specific goal and gain, which may be spiritual or health-related. Starvation is the involuntary absence of food, which eventually leads to suffering and even death. The former is usually done by people who have enough body fats stored to carry them through for a specific period. It is not recommended for underweight people and does not in any way lead to suffering and or death. When fasting, food is available, but the dieter chooses to do without it for some hours, days, and even weeks, depending on how long they can go without eating. You may choose to start or stop fasting at any time.

Even though intermittent fasting is currently gaining widespread recognition across the globe, it is not as new as people may realize. Fasting has been in existence for centuries now. It is probably the most potent and oldest dietary intervention in the history of man; however, it has been overlooked and relegated. To get the best results out of this method, you should familiarize yourself with everything there is to know about it.

How Intermittent Fasting Works for Weight Loss

When you engage in intermittent fasting, your body begins to use its stored fat as a source of energy. It is the reason that you can typically function for hours without food. This means that, when you fast, your body burns excess fat and keeps you from feeling hungry. The fact is that fasting and eating are opposite of each other. At any point, you can choose to either eat or fast. When you eat, your body gets more energy than it actually needs, while the insulin level rises immediately. With the help of insulin, the excess fat in the body gets stored away to be used at a later time. It also allows the storage of carbohydrates into individual glucose units, which are linked with long-chain glycogen, which is later stored in the liver. For biological reasons, there is hardly enough space in the liver to store glycogen. Once the limit is reached, therefore, the body automatically transforms excess glucose into fat. This process is known as de novo lipogenesis, which means "making new fat." While some of the newly created fat is stored in the liver, others get deposited in other parts of the body. Although this is a complicated process, there is absolutely no limit to the amount of fat that can be produced naturally.

During intermittent fasting, there is a drastic fall in the level of insulin in your body, thus sending a signal to your entire system to notify your body parts of the scarcity of energy from food. This makes you experience a drop in the level of blood glucose, forcing the body to go to the storage facilities to get energized. Glycogen, which is the most accessible source of energy, is in limited supply. It can only last for about 24 to 36 hours. Once the stored glycogen is exhausted, your body is then forced to break down the stored fat to get energy. This means that your body survives in either the fed state, which is the insulin-high state, or the fasted state, which is the insulin-low state. The former contributes to weight gain because if, say, if you spend your entire day eating, there will be no room for the body to burn fat from the stored reserves. It is necessary for your body to strike a balance between the fed state and the fasted state so that it can burn stored fat and allow you to lose weight. This is precisely what intermittent fasting does, and there is absolutely nothing wrong with it. As mentioned above, it is how our bodies are wired. If you continue to eat without resting, the body will always have glycogen to use. This causes it to keep storing what you eat as fat until you have nothing to eat. That's the only time when it can burn the excess fat. Without ever being in the fasted state, there will never be a need for your body to consume stored fat so you will keep gaining weight.

Although some benefits come with intermittent fasting, aside from religious purposes, weight loss is the main reason why people fast. While fasting, you eat fewer meals, leading to an automatic reduction in the level of calories. It also changes the levels of hormones that aid in weight loss. It causes an increase in the level of fat-burning hormones norepinephrine or noradrenaline. These changes in hormones contribute to the rise in the metabolic rate of the body by 3.6-14%. The caloric equation is also affected on both sides to create a balance by helping you during intermittent fasting by eating fewer calories while burning more of them. According to a study, this fast makes people lose muscle than other known standard methods (Gunnars, 2016). Eating large amounts of food during this period may increase your caloric level and have the opposite effect that you are aiming for.

Several benefits attached to intermittent fasting include, overall health improvement, increased brain condition, can reduce the risk of developing type 2 diabetes, cancer, and heart-related diseases.

Science Behind Intermittent Fasting

To dissect the science behind intermittent fasting, we will take a quick look at the history of the dietary pattern, which experts say dates back to as far as two million years ago. It is theorized to begin during the evolution of the genus homo, that we humans are evolved from, whom anthropologists believe to be hunters. This is how it worked at the time: when a band of hunters killed game that they found, it meant that they had a bounty of a calorie-rich diet. At the end of the feast, they were left to survive on herbs, cereal grains, and roots that had little to no calories at all. After agriculture was invented by humans about ten thousand years ago, there is now a predictable and surplus supply of calories. Fast forward to modern times, and us humans have been able to maximize survival capacity through a metabolic and biochemical food selection process in times of food-related crises, such as famines and scarcity of food. This is why humans now have tendencies of being plump and even obese. The reason behind the overweight trends, however, lies in the psychology of modern times. Our metabolic standpoint has become higher than when our ancestors had to survive on hunting and gathering to survive. Scientifically speaking, there have not been a significant amount of changes in the metabolic processes of Homo sapiens sapiens, which are geared towards conserving energy related to uneven caloric reserves. Due to food intake restrictions by our ancestors, the body developed a means to maintain its functions. This is essential for the body to adapt perfectly in times when you change your diet. Our modern world has made food varieties available, and we get to eat what we want anytime. In fact, many health practitioners have advised that people should spread their meals to 5 or 6 different times a day. The body sees this as a food surplus, which affects its ability to repair vital tissues that should slow down the aging process.

Consequently, the hormones charged with the responsibility of maintaining the physiological stability now resists changes in the set metabolic point. This is a phenomenon that is known to everyone who has ever gone on a diet. Also, theorists say that there is a problem with our gut flora, a community of microorganisms that live in the digestive tracts of humans and animals. According to experts, obesity causes a change in the gut where the new flora now promotes weight gain. This was probably not the case for people millennia ago.

Researchers from the Salk Institute went into an investigation and found that the method is not totally devoid of problems. According to a study done on mice, when food was withdrawn from them for 24 hours, 90% of the internal organs that are under the control of the circadian regulation ceased to function (Micheali, 2017). This isn't a remarkable feat as it is expected that the main metabolic organs will be primarily influenced by the amount of food. The study, however, also revealed that when the mice were placed on a high-fat diet, most of the organs became extremely active. As a result, the mice were reported to have become obese. This practically explains the science/mechanism behind intermittent fasting and feeding on a molecular level. There is still no conclusive research regarding the full extent of the benefits of intermittent fasting in humans.

Dr. Krysta Varady of the Illinois University in Chicago (2015) carried out a research on 86 obese women and 14 obese men (a total of 100 people), spread through three random groups, for a whole year. They were asked to observe alternate-day fasts, supplying them with 25% of their energy needs on fast days and 125% energy needs on eating days. As for calorie supplies, 75% of the caloric needs were supplied daily in some days, and there were no caloric restrictions at all on other days. This trial, however, involved phases of weight loss and gain for six months each. The result revealed that the alternate-day fasting did not produce superior adherence to weight loss, cardioprotection, or maintenance, as opposed to caloric restriction. Varady stated in an interview that the efficacy of intermittent fasting does not lay in any adaptation theory of evolution as propagated by historians or a complicated genetic, molecular mechanism. It rather lies in tricking/training your mind and body to eat less. As a result of weight loss, the body gets all the metabolic benefits. This simply means that the method works not because of what goes on within us scientifically but because of the food that we eat, which is mainly characterized by how we consume it.

Effects of Intermittent Fasting on Cells and Hormones

During fasting, the body is exposed to several cellular and molecular activities. It needs to adjust and make stored fats more accessible. Below are some of the things that happen in the body during intermittent fasting.

1. Increases human growth hormones

The level of growth hormones, which is multiplied as much as five times, shoots up. It improves the loss of fat and increases the gains of muscle mass.

2. Improves insulin sensitivity

When you fast, the levels of insulin in your body drops drastically while improving insulin sensitivity. The lower the insulin level is, the easier it is to access the fat that has been stored in your system.

3. Repairs cells

When you are fasting, the body automatically initiates a process called autophagy that repairs cells. The digestion of old and dysfunctional proteins that have been stored inside the cell also takes place.

4. Expresses genes

The genes that are related to longevity also undergo some changes and experience protection against diseases.

5. Reduces inflammation

Some studies have noted a drastic reduction in some inflammation markers, which are vital contributors to various chronic diseases.

6. Prevents cancer

According to a study on animals, intermittent fasting can be a great contributor to the reduction or prevention of cancer (Gunnars, 2016).

7. Improves brain health

The brain hormone BDNF is increased by intermittent fasting, leading to the growth of new nerve cells. It also contributes to protecting against Alzheimer's disease.

8. Promotes anti-aging

Studies say that intermittent fasting can increase the lifespan of rats that have been used in some research. It showed that the rats that were placed on the fast had chances of living 80% longer.

Methods of Intermittent Fasting

Thankfully, the intermittent fast is a natural regimen that can be done in whichever way you want. For more extended fasting periods, it is advised that the fast should be done under the supervision of a health practitioner. On a general note, shorter fasts are the most commonly practiced. There are several ways that you can try fasting intermittently, but you are expected to split days or weeks into periods of both eating and fasting on all of them. During the fasting periods, though, you may either eat very little or eat nothing at all.

The most popular fasting methods are:

16/8 Method

This technique also called the Lean Gains protocol. You are required to fast for 16 hours. It is sometimes also known as the 8-hour eating window. Here, all your meals are eaten within 8 hours, while you avoid food of any kind in the remaining 16 hours. With this method, you simply skip breakfast, eat the other meals within the 8-hour window, and fast for the rest of the day. Although most people do not eat in the morning, others prefer to skip dinner. Typically, the technique involves eating two to three meals daily. On this fast, you can drink as many zero-calorie beverages as you want.

Eat-Stop-Eat

This fasting method entails that you should not eat anything for 24 hours twice a week. It is a technique that has been introduced by Brad Pilon. Without any form of restrictions, the only rule is that you must fast for 24 hours and that the fasting must not be done on two consecutive days. It is not advisable for people who are not used to skipping meals. It can be absolutely impossible for some people to stay away from foods for 24 hours. They tend to feel extremely hungry during that period, to the extent that these folks might become irritable and unable to function normally.

Warrior Diet

This is a fasting method introduced by Ori Hofmekler, and it entails that people should eat a small amount of food within 20 hours daily. This method requires you to eat all of your meals in the remaining 24 hours of the day. This, however, may not be a simple technique to try as the consumption of a large amount of food may not settle well with your stomach. It is regarded as the most extreme fasting method and cannot be recommended to people who are barely getting used to fasting.

Alternate-Day Fasting (5/2 Method)

The technique is used to improve blood sugar, calorie, and cholesterol levels by fasting on alternate days. With the 5/2 method, you're expected to eat 500 to 600 calories on two non-consecutive days every week. For some people, an extra day is added every week. For the remaining days of the week, the individual should merely consume the same number of calories that he or she has burned during the day. The result is that there will be a deficiency in calories over time so that you begin to lose weight.

Exercising During Intermittent Fasting

If you are fasting and still want to continue your workout routines, there are some things you must consider before doing so. Those who are fasting to lose weight, the good news is that when fasting and exercise are combined, you have a higher possibility of dissolving more fats. While some research says that combining fasting and exercise affects the biochemistry and metabolism of the muscles that are linked with insulin sensitivity and the control of blood sugar levels, others support exercising immediately after eating before the occurrence of digestion and absorption. This is said to be essential for people suffering from type 2 diabetes and metabolic syndrome. The good thing about fasting is that glycogen is likely depleted during fasting so you will burn more fat to fuel your exercise. Other studies have countered this research, though, claiming that people do not burn more by exercising on an empty stomach. If you think that exercising while fasting is a good idea, you may want to consider some of its downsides (Weatherspoon, 2018).

Working out and fasting at the same time can lead to the loss of muscles. Because of that, you may be able to maintain your muscles, but you cannot gain more. Your body can break down tissues and use their protein as energy during intermittent fasting. This means is that you will have limited power to work out as hard or perform as well as you usually do on a regular diet. There is also a chance of you falling or hitting a wall. Another theory states that the body reduces its calories and energy, so it may end up slowing down your metabolic processes.

Tips for Combining Intermittent Fasting with Exercise

If you are convinced that your body genuinely needs a combination of intermittent fasting and exercise, here are some things you may want to try to get the best out of both regimens.

1. Think about timing critically

Christopher Shuff (2018), a dietician, says that there are three things to consider in order to make workout effective while fasting. He states that you should consider whether he or she wants to exercise during, before or after the fueling window. One of the most common methods of combining exercise with intermittent fasting is the Lean Gains 16:8 protocol. For someone who can function well when exercising on an empty stomach, working out before the timeframe is an ideal option. If you do not like to work out on an empty stomach, doing it during the window is best. This is also a good option because you get to tap into all the post-workout nutrition. Shuff, however, explains that exercising while fasting is beneficial when it comes to recovery and performance. Working out after the window, therefore, is for those who prefer to work out with a satiated stomach but do not have the chance to do so during the eating period.

2. Select workout types based on your macros

According to experts, it is crucial to pay attention to the macronutrients that you eat during the day before and after your workout session. For example, having a high amount of carbohydrates is essential for strength training, while eating a small number of carbs can be acceptable when you are doing high-intensity interval training (HIIT).

3. Build or maintain muscles

You should build or keep muscles by eating the right foods after exercising. The best option for the individuals who wish to combine working out with intermittent fasting is to time the fitness periods so that they correlate with eating periods to ensure that nutrition levels are at their peak. For someone who lifts heavy weights, it is a good idea to eat protein after a workout session to aid in muscle regeneration. It is advised to consume approximately 20 grams of protein within 30 minutes post-workout.

As you may already know, the success of any exercise or weight-loss regimen depends on its safety and sustainability over time. If you intend to lose weight while maintaining your fitness level during intermittent fasting, you should try to stay in the safe zone as much as possible.

- **Eat a meal close to your workout**: Having your meal at a time when your moderate or high-intensity exercise is close is very important. By doing so, there will be glycogen available for your body to tap into to gain energy.

- **Stay hydrated**: Always keep in mind that even if you are fasting, it does not mean that you should avoid drinking water. As a matter of fact, it is during this time that you need more water than ever. Therefore, you are advised to drink lots of water when fasting, and even more so when you fast and exercise simultaneously.

- **Keep your electrolytes up**: Be mindful of sports drinks during workouts because most of them are high in sugar. You should try to avoid them as much as you can. A good substitute for such beverages is coconut water, which is a high-caloric source of hydration. While it replenishes the electrolytes in your body, it also provides a low amount of calories.

- **Combine low-intensity workouts with short workout time**: If you are engaging in the 24-hour intermittent fast, try to carry out low-intensity workouts, such as restorative yoga and walking. When doing the other types, you may stick with regular exercise routines.

- **Listen to your body**: Finally, the best thing to do when working out during an intermittent fast is to listen to your body. You will know when you have reached your limit and can no longer push forward further. If, for example, you begin to feel weak or dizzy, it is a clear sign that you have either become dehydrated or experienced a drop in your blood sugar level. In cases like this, you are advised to drink electrolytes immediately and then eat a well-balanced meal as soon as possible.

In a nutshell, while the combination of intermittent fasting and exercise may be an excellent idea for some people, it's not ideal for others who need to stay away from any strenuous activity while fasting. Whatever the situation may be, it is always good to check with a healthcare expert before engaging in any exercise or nutritional activity.

Enjoying this book so far? I'd love it for you to share your thoughts and post a quick review on Amazon!

Chapter 7: Benefits of Intermittent Fasting

Weight Loss

Considering many people who go on the fast do so for the sole purpose of losing weight, this is the most popular benefit of intermittent fasting. The popularity of the method has been gaining more ground in recent years as a result of its efficacy in promoting weight loss. Fasting pushes the body to shed a few pounds by bringing down insulin levels (a hormone that allows cells to take in glucose). Typically, the system breaks carbohydrates down to glucose, which is later used by cells for energy, or converted into fat and stored in the body for future use. During the times when you are not eating, there is usually a drop in the levels of insulin. The depleting insulin levels cause cells to release the stored glucose as energy. The repetition of this process, which takes place during intermittent fasting, may lead to the loss of weight. Not to mention, the consumption of a fewer amount of calories can cause a reduction in weight. Though it may not be more effective than other traditional techniques that are based on caloric restrictions, intermittent fasting is doable for people who want to start shedding some pounds.

Reduction in the Risk Type 2 Diabetes

Together with its weight loss benefits, intermittent fasting is also useful when it comes to reducing the risk of having or worsening type 2 diabetes. To be specific, it influences other factors that are linked to the condition.

According to health experts, obesity is one of the things that contribute to the development of type 2 diabetes. A 2014 study that has been published in the journal called Translation Research has stated that intermittent fasting can lower blood glucose and insulin levels in people who are at the risk of developing diabetes. Other researches back it up by claiming that fasting is a promising therapy for weight loss and diabetes (Kandola, 2018).

When further studies were conducted to adults who suffer from obesity, it was discovered that there were reductions in diabetes markers (such as sensitivity to insulin), so experts believe that the fast can be useful in the reduction of the disease among this group. On the contrary, a 2018 research conducted on rats showed that intermittent fasting could be capable of increasing the risk of diabetes (Ana, 2018). By tracking the well-being of rodents for three months, it later came out that despite the reduction in weight and food eaten, the abdominal fat tissue increased while the muscle structure decreased - a clear sign of the body not making proper use of insulin. All of these are risk factors of type 2 diabetes (Kandola, 2018). This study, therefore, gives rise to the need for it to be replicated in humans to find out if the results apply to us as well.

Brain Health

As people get older, there is a limited flow of blood to the brain. Neurons shrink, and there is a decline in the amount of brain volume. Luckily, intermittent fasting is capable of stalling the aging process by improving the alertness and overall mental health of humans. Some benefits of intermittent fasting to the brain are:

1. Lowering the risk of brain diseases

Intermittent fasting is capable of boosting the health of your mind by reducing the risk of neurodegenerative diseases such as Alzheimer's and Parkinson's. It is imperative when it comes to the prevention of diabetes and obesity, considering both conditions contribute to the development of Alzheimer's disease.

2. Promotes autophagy and prevents neural degeneration

Another benefit of intermittent fasting is that it assists the brain in preventing the degeneration of nerve cells. According to a 2003 study, the neurons in the brain can be protected against excitotoxic stress, which later leads to neural death, thanks to intermittent fasting (Moodie). Autophagy, which is the process that the brain goes through to get rid of damaged cells and produce new ones, is also boosted by the method. This allows the body to defend itself against various illnesses naturally.

3. Improves memory

It has also been found that intermittent fasting is capable of boosting learning and memory retention. This is another potent protection against neurodegenerative diseases. Using their ability to recall words, a study carried out in 50 aged people found a boost of memory after getting placed on caloric restriction for three months (Moodie, n.d.).

4. Alleviates depression

Intermittent fasting may also be beneficial for people who deal with mood disorders like depression. According to research in 2013, depressed individuals reported improvements in mental alertness and mood and experienced a sense of peace when they fasted (Moodie).

Longevity

Studies have proven that intermittent fasting helps to guard the body against terminal diseases. Someone devoid of cancer, cardiovascular disease, or diabetes, therefore, is bound to live longer.

1. Lowering cholesterol levels

A study that was carried out in 2010 showed that the overweight women who fasted intermittently showed improvements in some risk factors for chronic diseases (Moodie, n.d.). This includes lowered cholesterol, reduced blood pressure, as well as decreased level of insulin resistance.

2. Slowing down cancer

When combined with chemotherapy, intermittent fasting is also capable of slowing down the progress of skin and other forms of cancer by increasing the level of tumor-infiltrating lymphocytes. These are the cells sent by the immune system to fight the tumor.

3. Making cells resistant

The manipulation of mitochondrial networks is also a way for intermittent fasting to improve your lifespan and slow down the aging process. Mitochondria is the powerhouse - the power generator - of a cell. For the cells to survive, they rely on this organ to provide all the energy they need. A study conducted by Harvard researchers in 2017, however, showed that fasting helped to keep the mitochondria networks together by keeping them healthy enough to process energy effectively. The latter is vital to aging and longevity.

Inflammation Reduction

We are confronted with inflammation in one way or another every day. This can take place if you kick a stone accidentally or get cut from a knife while preparing your family's dinner. It can be the result of a fungus that triggers allergies. When inflammation graduates to a chronic condition, it can lead to excess belly fats and weight gain.

Intermittent fasting has proven to be a handy tool to combat this situation. By not eating, the body produces an anti-inflammatory effect on the body's neurological and immune systems. This is a process that can't happen when you consume meals that are high in carbohydrates. When combined with the keto diet, intermittent fasting can help rid the body of inflammation and its effects.

Immune Regulation

Intermittent fasting forces the body's immune system to perform in peak condition. The majority of the body's energy will help fight off disease. Two major cytokines foster vital inflammatory responses: interleukin-6 and tumor necrosis factor alpha. When you fast, you restrict the release of such molecules.

When you fast intermittently and drink more water and other cleansing beverages, the effect is usually superb. The reason is that this activity cleanses your digestive system, which reduces your gut microbes that affect your immune system.

Insulin Sensitivity Enhancement

Intermittent fasting is a useful tool to improve cellular insulin sensitivity. This allows the body to make effective use of insulin so that it requires less of this chemical after eating. With reduced demand for insulin, the inflammation level reduces and bumps up the body's HGH levels. Insulin and human growth hormone (HGH) work in diverse ways in the body. The former triggers the storage of energy while boosting cellular division and inflammation. The primary assignment of the latter is to encourage tissue repair while at the same time. Between the two, insulin is more valuable. When we consume foods that are rich in starch and carbs, insulin is required to suppress the level of HGH.

During periods of food scarcity, the sensitivity of the body's cell membrane to insulin increases. This is expected - and quite significant - because it makes the body utilize every chunk of food that goes in it. When there is more than enough food, on the other hand, the opposite happens. The body, in a bid to dodge the stress of excessive calorie intake, reduces its sensitivity to insulin. It leads to an increase in insulin level, which then results in excess body fats, inflammatory conditions, and oxidative stress.

Intermittent Fasting and Chronic Diseases

Intermittent fasting has been known to bring about splendid improvements in patients and victims of chronic autoimmune diseases, such as Crohn's, ulcerative colitis, rheumatoid arthritis, and systemic lupus. This is because intermittent fasting tends to reduce the effect of inflammation that causes these illnesses and leads to a normal function of the body's immune system.

Cancer cells, for instance, contains between ten and seventy other insulin receptors more than the average cell. This is the result of the breakdown of sugar, which serves as the body's energy source. When you are fasting intermittently, the body does not get the fuel (sugar) it requires for this disintegration. Thus, cells with free radicals can be destroyed.

While there is a lot of research being conducted regarding the effects of intermittent fasting, experts say that the results are yet to be conclusive. It may take a while before doctors can recommend this technique for clinical use. There is not enough evidence to support some of the claims made by propagators of the theory. It is an established fact that fasting can contribute to weight loss. Also, although many experiments have been carried out on animals, based on the hypothesis of the intermittent fast, most of these researches are yet to be transitioned from animals to humans.

Chapter 7: Intermittent Fasting in Men vs. Women

While it is all right for everyone to observe intermittent fasting, some studies have shown that the results of the fast may not be the same in some women as it is in men. According to research, controlling the blood sugar became more difficult for the females than the males three weeks after they began fasting intermittently (Coyle, 2018). There are also many claims made by women, who believe that their menstrual cycle had changed when they started intermittent fasting. These shifts are tied to the sensitivity of the female population to calorie restrictions.

When there is a low level of calorie due to long hours of fasting or frequent fasting, a part of the brain, which is known as the hypothalamus, is affected. This disrupts the hormone that releases gonadotropin. This hormone further releases two reproductive hormones, which are known as the luteinizing hormone (LH) and the follicle-stimulating hormone (FSH). When there is a breach of communication between these hormones and the ovaries, women run the risk of experiencing irregular menstruations, poor bone health, infertility, and other health complications. Though studies in animals have not been replicated in humans, a research carried out on rats showed that they experienced a reduction in the size of their ovaries when they were placed on three to six months of alternate-day fasting. Irregular reproductive cycles were also some of the side effects of the fast in female rats (Coyle, 2018). These are several reasons why it is advised for women to consider a modified approach to intermittent fastings, such as shorter fasting periods and fewer fasting days. In short, fasting methods that women follow should be less intense than their male counterparts. It is important to note that metabolism and the human reproductive system are deeply interwoven. When a woman misses her period, it is evident that there has been some form of disturbance in her hormones. The hormones that affect a woman's reproductive health are not only restricted to the sex hormones. The ones that store fat as well as in burning it contributes to that process. Because of this, any hormonal imbalance that a woman may experience will likely reflect in her reproductive system.

The less frequent eating pattern that is characterized by intermittent fasting means that you eat less protein. The lack of protein causes negative impacts on women's fertility rate. Stress is your system's antagonist as it raises your cortisol levels and inhibits the production of gonadotropin-releasing hormone, which hinders the ovaries from generating estrogen and progesterone. In truth, the latter is usually converted to cortisol during periods of stress to help the body to cope. This may either prevent weight loss or contribute to weight gain. The singular fact that you eat little food during the fasting stresses out the body as well.

In general, anything capable of affecting reproductive health will also affect weight management, fitness, and well-being, as well as your overall health. If you think intermittent fasting is becoming stressful, you may want to consider that it probably isn't suitable for you. These are some of the reasons why women are advised to try the less stressful versions of the method and take notes of the way their body responds to it.

During the fasting period, pay close attention to the following signs and discontinue the fast if you develop any of them: menstrual irregularities, insomnia, hair loss, slow recovery after injury, acne/rashes, low libido, mood swings, palpitations, sluggish digestion, reduced tolerance to stress, or feeling cold constantly. Intermittent fasting is not recommended to anyone pregnant, suffering or recovering from an eating disorder, battling insomnia, on medication for a chronic condition, under severe stress, depressed, or dealing with any form of severe illness, unless under the direct supervision of a medical professional.

Intermittent Fasting Modifications for Women

If you wish to attempt to try intermittent fasting as a woman, there are some alterations you should make to the plan to make it less strict compared to the standard versions that work for men. While doing this, she will need to consider hunger signals. She can be sure that they are not caused by simple eating habits or boredom; whenever her body indicates the need for food, it is not just merely showing the sign for the fun of it. Chances are, it needs something important, and the consequences of turning a blind eye to it may not be pleasant. Here are some of the things that women can do to make intermittent fasting suitable for them.

Eat Healthy Fats

As you already know, fat isn't something that should be avoided. Essential fatty acids must be part of your diet, in fact, to fight inflammation and improve mental health, among others. When you choose to eat healthy fats, i.e., grass-fed butter, and coconut oil, not only will there be significant work in progress within the body, but there will also be a feeling of satisfaction. You may choose to rely solely on fats during this time without fear of interrupting the body's state of ketosis since you will surely receive enough calories even during this brief eating period.

Choose Low-Impact Foods

Intermittent fasting allows the digestive tract to recuperate and rebuild. This can be supported and given a boost when you choose to consume low-impact foods instead of subjecting yourself to a complete fast. Some common foods that suit this purpose are steamed vegetables, nutritionally rich green powder, and fruits.

Reduce Your Fasting Period

While sleeping, the body naturally goes into a fasting period. This gets broken in the morning once you wake up. This nightly fast can be extended for longer hours, possibly until noon, instead of farther into the day. This way, you will be giving your body a chance to ease the fast into your daily routine without putting in more effort or going through more stress.

Whether you are one of those women whom intermittent fasting works for, or you belong to the group needs to alter their habits drastically, you should find other ways to apply the fasting principles. By paying attention to your body's signals, you will be able to prepare for potential health risks ahead of time. This enables you to look for the best options for your body while staying away from things that may be detrimental to your overall well-being. Like every other dietary program, you should always keep a close watch at methods that work for you as an individual. We have already covered that there is no one-size-fits-all approach to dieting. The fact that a particular method is beneficial for other women does not necessarily mean that it will work in the same way for you.

Chapter 8: Intermittent Fasting and Ketogenic Diet

Intermittent fasting and the ketogenic diet are two of the most recent trends among the health-conscious crowd. Many benefits come from both programs, and many types of research have been done to back them up. While they are best known for controlling weight, that's not all that these two techniques can do. With the growing popularity surrounding these trends, many people are curious as to if these weight-loss methods can be implemented together without possible side effects. The idea of combining both practices is welcome but not absolutely necessary.

If you are one of those individuals who is considering combining both practices, there is good news for you: you can easily follow both of them simultaneously without having to face severe consequences.

Some of the reasons why following the keto diet and intermittent fasting can be right for you are:

1. It makes it easier for your body to reach ketosis.

Adding fasting to your regimen may jumpstart the process of ketosis. This is because the body maintains a balance of energy by shifting its source of fuel from carbs to fat, which is the specific premise of the keto diet. When you fast, your insulin and glycogen levels drop and trigger the burning of fats automatically to maintain enough energy. The combination of both techniques is, therefore, suitable for those people who cannot reach ketosis when only following the ketogenic diet. It may be quicker for your body to enter ketosis when you combine a keto diet with intermittent fasting than merely doing either individually.

2. You may not experience cravings.

When on a keto diet, there is no fear of fat spiking your blood sugar levels. After all, we know by now that fat stabilizes blood sugar. This is so effective that it has been recorded to cure individuals with type 2 diabetes and get them totally off of medication. Combining keto diet and fasting can reduce your blood sugar level without causing you to feel uncomfortable. You can now say goodbye to programs that make you feel awkward with high-carb fasting and induced cravings, fatigue, and mood swings.

3. It helps suppress your hunger.

The ketogenic diet is also very useful in keeping hunger at bay. The liver turns fat stores into ketone energy bundles while you are on the plan. These organic compounds are sent as fuel through the bloodstream. As a result, the ghrelin levels get suppressed during the ketogenic diet. Ghrelin, the primary hunger hormone of the body is suppressed to a minimal level, even when there is no food in your system. Thanks to them, you may not be as hungry as you usually are when you are on a regular weight-loss journey. This causes you to go for hours without feeling famished. That is a definite advantage while you are intermittent fasting. You can then stay on the fast for more extended periods to assist your body in shedding even more pounds.

4. It leads to more fat loss.

You are more likely to burn fat when you combine the fast and the diet than when you are on the diet alone. Simply because intermittent fasting boosts metabolism by promoting thermogenesis or heat production. During thermogenesis, the body automatically begins to search out those stubborn fat stores that are ordinarily inaccessible to start turning those deposits into energy. It is no longer new that intermittent fasting is capable of reducing excess body fat. According to a study that was carried out in 34 resistance-trained men for eight weeks, the ones who practiced the 16:8 fasting method lost approximately 14% more body fat than those who followed the regular dietary pattern. In the same light, the men who supported the low-carb diet lost about 3.3 kilograms (7.3 lbs) of fat mass than the people who followed the proper low-calorie diet (Kubala, 2018). Intermittent fasting also preserves muscle mass when you are losing weight, as well as improving your energy level. This is helpful to those keto dieters who are looking for ways to enhance their athletic performance while continuing to drop some unwanted extra weight.

5. It helps you avoid the side effects of ketosis.

The ketogenic diet can make your fasting periods more natural and more manageable than ever before. For example, when you consume a high amount of carbohydrates while fasting, the fast will cause you to be uncomfortable as your body struggles to make the switch between glucose and ketones for fuel. Eating keto meals during fasting, however, will allow your system to run on ketones whenever you want it to.

If you are either not used to the keto diet or merely starting back up after a break, it is advisable for you to start your journey again with intermittent fasting. This will help you to avoid some of the adverse side effects that you might experience during the early stages of the program, particularly the keto flu. Which you already know is brought on as a result in the drop of glucose levels in the blood while it is switching its use from regular carbohydrates and proteins as their source of energy to ketones from fat.

6. It helps autophagy to work better.

Intermittent fasting activates something called autophagy in the body. This is a state where the body eats its own cells and tissues in an attempt to keep the body healthy. Through this process, the body cleanses itself by getting rid of harmful and toxic substances and recycles damaged proteins. Autophagy operations happen under two conditions: 1) when the body is starved, and 2) when there are restrictions in protein and carbohydrate levels. Because both of these processes take place in both ketogenic dieting and intermittent fasting, their combination will help you reap all the benefits of autophagy healthily and efficiently.

For the majority of people, combining intermittent fasting and the keto diet is a perfectly safe and healthy thing to do. However, as mentioned in other chapters, we want to emphasize that it might not be suitable for everyone. Pregnant women and those who have suffered from an eating disorder are advised to stay away from intermittent fasting. As well as those individuals who are dealing with diabetes or heart-related diseases should consult their doctor before subjecting themselves to either method of losing weight.

Although it might be helpful for some people to combine both practices, you should first find out if it is compatible with your system to know if it's even worth pursuing or not. Besides the possibility of following both techniques being too risky health-wise for some, others may begin to experience adverse side effects, such as overeating during non-fasting days, irritability, and even fatigue. You should always remember that although intermittent fasting is capable of making you reach ketosis faster, you do not really need it to reach ketosis. Keto dieting alone will allow you to enter that metabolic state. The most important adjustment for a healthier lifestyle is a well-rounded low-carb diet, which is found by following the ketogenic diet.

If you have decided to take part in the two simultaneously, you should do so when you are already in a state of ketosis. This will make fasting more manageable for you to cope with as your body is already making use of fat as an energy source, and you do not need to have extra carbohydrates to fuel your system. You should also be careful with choosing the fasting method that will suit your needs and doesn't push you beyond your limits.

Tips for a Successful Keto and Fasting Plan

At this point, we figure that you have most likely decided to combine the keto diet and intermittent fasting. If you wish to go the extra mile to achieve these positive results, you can combine the two; however, as with every new health experience of this nature, you should consult your doctor before you begin. Before you start on this path, though, here are some guidelines that you should consider incorporating into your plan to achieve the best results.

1. Eat enough

Naturally, intermittent fasting ensures that you eat less during the day. Regardless of that, try to continue to eat healthy keto-friendly foods to help your system stay away from deficits and metabolic difficulties. With the help of an app or website, you can track the ideal caloric level for your body, as well as your essential macronutrients for each day. These will also help you monitor them to ensure that you are getting enough nutrients daily. It is necessary to get a sufficient amount of fats during the fasting period from either seed, olive oil, or avocado. Also, you should add protein sources, as well as some low-carb vegetables to incorporate fiber into your diet.

2. Measure your ketone levels

Although fasting will help you stay in ketosis for a more extended period, make sure that you are not eating too many carbs or anything capable of jolting you out of ketosis. It is imperative for you to keep track of your ketone level to guarantee that you are always in this metabolic state.

3. Start with shorter fasting windows

If you are combining a keto diet and intermittent fasting, the best way to go about it is, to start off with short fasting windows. This allows you to then build them up as you get used to the practice and make it into a routine. Using the keto diet as a base is one of the most widely practiced strategies out there. With the keto diet as a guide, you can also do the 24-hour fast and eat a ketogenic meal once a day. Adding the 16:8 fasting method to your plan is also an excellent decision. You fast for 16 hours in a day and only consume your keto-friendly meals during the eight-hour window.

4. Plan your meals

The focal point of the keto diet is the need to eat the proper amount of fats daily. Intermittent fasting, on the other hand, focuses on the reduction of the number of times you eat every day. Combining both practices consist of you putting in extra effort by paying more attention to not just what you eat but how you eat as well. The ideal approach is to plan your meals and snacks more than you did ordinarily.

5. Know the facts

When you are combining two different plans, it is vital to keep a few points in mind to help you determine if you should continue with it and ensure that you will achieve success.

a. Restrictive dietary patterns do not lead to weight loss.

If you are thinking of ways to maintain a healthy lifestyle, you should first consider the possibility of avoiding processed foods, reducing the intake of calories, and cutting added sugar and carbohydrate sources like bread, pasta, baked goods, and so on. You should also increase your physical activities. For someone who wants to lose weight, it is not necessary to follow a restrictive dietary pattern. Try other opportunities and keep the restrictive nutritional habits such as intermittent fasting and keto diet as your last resort.

b. Intermittent fasting and the keto diet are not recommended for everyone.

We have said this numerous times because it is important. Although the practice of combining intermittent fasting and the keto diet is relatively safe for most people, it is not recommended for everybody. Therefore, before you get started with both programs, make sure that it will not be detrimental to your health by figuring out if you belong to a group of people for whom the diet is applicable for.

> c. There are no conclusive reports to support both plans yet.

For what it's worth, the combination of the keto diet and intermittent fasting does not have strong scientific backings yet. Summer Yule, a registered dietician, once said that she will not recommend the combo because there is no research on humans that speak of its benefits.

6. Do not become overwhelmed

Jumping into the keto diet and intermittent fasting may be overwhelming and too much for you to handle. To avoid feeling like that, you should either begin with one before trying the other or vice versa. This way, your body should have adjusted to one before experimenting by adding the other.

Tips on Getting Comfortable With Intermittent Fasting

We thought that it would be significant to give you specific suggestions if you decide to try out intermittent fasting. Fasting can be tedious for some people, and we aim to help you ease into it gradually.

- Water is critical whenever you are fasting, even in days when you will be eating. Be sure to drink at least 8 glasses of water per day.
- It is vital to stay busy while on your fast. Being idle will cause the program to weigh heavily on you and may tempt you to give up.
- Whenever you decide to fast, make sure that critical tasks are done before the early hours of the day. A night before your fast, plan your day and work on a to-do list (if possible). Besides, all important tasks should be done in the hours after breakfast to keep your mind occupied.
- To see a noticeable result with your efforts, you need to give yourself time. Wait for at least three weeks before deciding if your aim is yielding anything tangible or not. Stay on the program consistently in that period as well to be able to come to a conclusion.

- As you proceed with the fast, monitor

your progress. The best way to do this is by taking pictures. When you associate yourself with the progress that you are making, then it will be easier to decide if your body is changing for the better or not. It is not just about the scale alone, but how you feel.

- Before starting either keto dieting or intermittent fasting, the involvement of your doctor is vital. He or she is in the best position to decide if it is beneficial for you.
- For people who want to attempt intermittent fasting, the best approach is to grow into it. You can do this by delaying breakfast gradually, depending on the type of fats you are going for. You can shift your first meal to either 11 A.M. or noon.
- As soon as you get out of bed every day, drink a glass of water. We recommend adding mint leaves or sliced lemon to it. This will give the extra beverage flavor and make it quite nutritious.
- If you wish to try the alternate-day fasting, we recommend that you limit this to two times a week. Going for

more days than that will just force your body to function too hard.

- It is essential to stick to healthy meals only. Choose the recommended keto meal plans that we have analyzed in the earlier part of this book, as a guide. Also, eat more fruits and vegetables when you are not fasting.
- Be sure not to live a boring life due to this lifestyle. Go out and have fun; don't pass on a night out with your girlfriends or buddies in the name of fasting. Nevertheless, you should watch what you eat.
- Avoid junk, fast, and processed foods at all costs. These are not healthy and will cancel out the expected results you aim for.
- Motivate yourself by having visual reminders of why you are doing this, e.g., stickers with messages in strategic places of the house. This way, you get to stay on track and keep inspired to continue. These are great, especially when a hunger pang comes at you with everything in its arsenal.
- We need you to understand that breakfast is not the most important

meal of the day. Your first meal is. So, make it delicious, nutritious, healthy, and keto-friendly.

Though intermittent fasting may seem uncomfortable at the beginning, keep going and don't give up on it. Give yourself enough time to adjust, your body will get used to fasting, and you will soon discover you no longer feel as hungry between feeding periods as you used to be. While fasting does not necessarily have to be a part of the ketogenic diet, it is absolutely possible to combine the two. If you wish to get the best out of them, it is essential for you to put in some effort to use them in the best ways possible.

Some Avoidable Mistakes

When you are on a keto diet, it is vital to keep in mind that the elimination of carbs for a high-fat diet is not a permanent change. Even though there is no adequate research to support the dangers of staying on a keto diet for a very long time, suggestions are pointing to the fact that continuing on ketosis for months on end may result in kidney stones, liver problems, osteoporosis, and high cholesterol. This is the reason why most experts advise people to remain on a keto diet for only three to six months at the most and then reintroduce carbs on certain days in specific intervals.

As for fasting, you should realize that you do not have to fast every day to procure all its benefits. As a matter of fact, subjecting yourself to fasting daily will make you weak, fatigued, and irritable. The focus should be on eating ketogenic meals first before you add fasting to your routine later. Being flexible will help you sustain the keto diet and intermittent fasting lifestyle for a more extended period.

On a final note, you should not make the mistake of ignoring those subtle or apparent signals that are sent by your body. If you are having some issues, consider increasing your carbohydrate and caloric intake a little bit. You can reduce the number of your fasting days every week as well. If that still is not helping and you feel sluggish, fatigued, or weak at any point, make sure to consult your physician, again, before continuing on with the programs.

Conclusion

Now that we have come to the end of this fantastic journey, we really do hope that you have enjoyed every bit of this ride as much as we have. At this point, we believe that you are fully equipped and for your own weight-loss journey while setting your sights on all the other health benefits that come with the two methods that have been discussed in this book.

If you have chosen to make use of the ketogenic diet as your guide for losing weight, pay attention to our tips and tricks so that you will not find yourself running into more trouble than you bargained for. While there are a lot of perks that come with this program, there are also possible dangers that might threaten your health in the long run if proper care is not taken from the onset, as it boosts your chances of developing kidney stones, among other things.

You also need to keep in mind that it is not always easy to carry on with the diet for a long time after you have reached ketosis. Even if you have the willpower to do so, it is not advisable for you to be on the keto diet forever. It is also important to note that while you are advised to go on a high-fat diet during your ketogenic dieting period, there are good and bad fats that you are now aware of and you know how to avoid consuming those unhealthy sources of fat.

Intermittent fasting is another dependable weight-loss technique that can help you reach ketosis and lose weight. Most people have found that it is an easy way to maintain this metabolic process, and they combine it with a ketogenic diet to get better results. While there are experts who are all for the combination of these two strategies, others are not totally convinced about the need for this union and refuse to recommend it. These are some of the reasons why they are still continuing to conduct research on this. Even now, there is no conclusive study to back the claims of the propagators of the combination theory. It is, therefore, strongly advised that you should consult your doctor before you adopt any of the two methods mentioned above.

We hope that you will be able to make the best out of all this material as you continue to pursue a healthy and happy lifestyle. Good luck!

If you enjoyed this book or received value from it in any way, then I'd like to ask you for a favor: would you be kind enough to leave a review for this book on Amazon? It'd be greatly appreciated!

References

Axe, J. (2018). Should you pair keto with intermittent fasting? Retrieved from https://whatsgood.vitaminshoppe.com/keto-intermittent-fasting/

Better Health Channel. (n.d.). Heart disease and food. Retrieved from https://www.betterhealth.vic.gov.au/health/conditionsandtreatments/heart-disease-and-food

BMJ. (2016). High intake of saturated fats is linked to increased risk of heart disease. Retrieved from https://www.bmj.com/content/355/bmj.i6347

Bonassa, A., and Carpinelli, A. (2018). Intermittent fasting for three months decreases pancreatic islet mass and increases insulin resistance in Wistar rats. *Endocrine Abstracts. 56,* 519. doi: 10.1530/endoabs.56.P519

Butler, N., (2017). Can fat be good for you? Retrieved from https://www.medicalnewstoday.com/articles/141442.php

Butler, N., (2019). How to begin intermittent fasting? Retrieved from https://www.medicalnewstoday.com/articles/324882.php

Coyle, D., (2018). Intermittent fasting for women: A beginner's guide. Retrieved from https://www.healthline.com/nutrition/intermittent-fasting-for-women

D'Andrea Meira, I., et al. (2019). Ketogenic diet and epilepsy: What we know so far. *Frontiers in Neuroscience.* doi: 10.3389/fnins.2019.00005

Designed for disease: the link between local food environments and obesity and diabetes. http://www.policylink.org/sites/default/files/DESIGNEDFORDISEASE_FINAL.PDF

Diet Doc. (n.d.). What is the origin of the ketogenic diet? Retrieved from https://www.dietdoc.com/diet-tips/ketogenic-diet-origin/

Diet review: Ketogenic diet for weight loss. (n.d.). Retrieved from https://www.hsph.harvard.edu/nutritionsource/healthy-weight/diet-reviews/ketogenic-diet/

Eenfeldt, A., (2018). The keto flu, other keto side effects, and how to cure them. Retrieved from https://www.dietdoctor.com/low-carb/keto/flu-side-effects

Eenfeldt, A., (2019). Low-carb and keto side effects & how to cure them. Retrieved from https://www.dietdoctor.com/low-carb/side-effects#badbreath

Fung, J., (2019). Intermittent fasting for beginners. Retrieved from https://www.dietdoctor.com/intermittent-fasting

Gustin, A., (2018). Intermittent fasting and ket: Can you do them both? Retrieved from https://perfectketo.com/intermittent-fasting-and-keto/

Hardick, B., (2015). An intermittent fasting guide for men & women. Retrieved from https://www.drhardick.com/intermittent-fasting-men-vs-women

Harvard Health Publishing. (n.d.). Should you try the keto diet? Retrieved from https://www.health.harvard.edu/staying-healthy/should-you-try-the-keto-diet

Harvard Health Publishing. (2015). The truth about fats: The good, the bad, and the in-between. Retrieved from https://www.health.harvard.edu/staying-healthy/the-truth-about-fats-bad-and-good

Hazmic, H. (n.d.). Intermittent fasting on keto: how does it work? Retrieved from https://www.kissmyketo.com/blogs/foods-nutrition/intermittent-fasting-on-keto-how-does-it-work

Jhaveri, A., (2017). 19 keto lunches that will help you stick to your resolutions. Retrieved from: https://greatist.com/eat/keto-lunches-that-will-help-you-stick-to-your-resolutions

Kubala, J., (2018). A keto diet meal plan and menu that can transform your body. Retrieved from https://www.healthline.com/nutrition/keto-diet-meal-plan-and-menu#meal-plan

Kubala, J., (2018). Intermittent fasting and keto: Should you combine the two? Retrieved from https://www.healthline.com/nutrition/intermittent-fasting-and-keto

Kubala, J., (2018). The keto flu: Symptoms and how to get rid of it. Retrieved from https://www.healthline.com/nutrition/keto-flu-symptoms#how-long-it-lasts

Leiva, C., (2018). How to do the keto and intermittent fasting at the same time, according to experts. Retrieved from https://www.thisisinsider.com/keto-and-intermittent-fasting-same-time-2018-10

Lindberg, R., (2018). How to exercise safely during intermittent fasting. Retrieved from https://www.healthline.com/health/how-to-exercise-safely-intermittent-fasting#2

Madell, R., and Nall, R. (2018). Good fats, bad fats, and heart disease. Retrieved from https://www.healthline.com/health/heart-disease/good-fats-vs-bad-fats#polyunsaturated-fat

Mawer, R., (2018). The ketogenic diet: A detailed beginner's guide to keto. Retrieved from https://www.healthline.com/nutrition/ketogenic-diet-101#types

McNew, A. (n.d.). 51 keto breakfast recipes to help you burn fat. Retrieved from https://blog.paleohacks.com/keto-breakfast-recipes/#

Michaeli, D., (2017). What science has to say about intermittent fasting. Retrieved from https://thedoctorweighsin.com/what-science-has-to-say-about-intermittent-fasting/

Moodie, A. (n.d.). The incredible benefits of intermittent fasting. Retrieved from https://blog.bulletproof.com/intermittent-fasting-benefits/

Nessler, T., (2009). Water and Your Diet: Staying Slim and Regular With H2O. Retrieved from https://www.webmd.com/diet/features/water-for-weight-loss-diet#1

Occhipinti, M., (2018). What is the history and evolution of the keto diet? Retrieved from https://www.afpafitness.com/blog/what-is-the-history-and-evolution-of-the-keto-diet

Olsen, N., (2018). What are the benefits of intermittent fasting? Retrieved from https://www.medicalnewstoday.com/articles/323605.php

Perfect Keto. (n.d.). Calculate your keto macros in minutes. Retrieved from https://perfectketo.com/keto-macro-calculator/

Pinkerton, J., (2018). Tips for a successful keto diet. Retrieved from https://www.wellhappyandkind.com/blog/2017/12/18/tips-for-a-successful-keto-diet

Ruled.me (n.d.). The 10 best tips for keto diet success. Retrieved from https://www.ruled.me/the-10-best-tips-for-keto-diet-success/

Siim Land. (2018). Ketogenic fasting mimicking diet how to. Retrieved from https://siimland.com/ketogenic-fasting-mimicking-diet-how-to/

Thorpe, M., (2017). 10 solid reasons why yo-yo dieting is bad for you. Retrieved from https://www.healthline.com/nutrition/yo-yo-dieting#section11

Thrive/Strive. (n.d.). Keto dinners: 16 delicious low carb dinners to prepare tonight. Retrieved from https://thrivestrive.com/keto-dinner-ideas/

Wikipedia. (2019). Keytones. Retrieved from https://en.wikipedia.org/wiki/Ketone

Autophagy Fasting With Water for Beginners

How to Master the Art of Weight Loss and Discover the Amazing Diet Secrets Behind the Power of Fasting! Lose Weight, Live Healthy, and Feel Younger!

Jason Berg   Eric Fung

Introduction

Autophagy ranks high among the most popular methods of weight management and healthy living, and this process is termed autophagy for a reason. Most people who have tried it can relate the benefits they have derived and the ways it has improved their life. But then, what is autophagy?

Do you suffer from recurrent body pains? Are you easily prone to illness, or do you find it difficult to shed some weight? Then, all you need to do is to acquire more knowledge of autophagy and the fasting processed involved.

This book will enlighten you on what autophagy is all about, the benefits associated with it and many more.

- Here is a clue of what lies ahead:

- All about autophagy; how it works, how to induce it, and its benefits

- Benefits and side effects of fasting, and precautions to take when fasting

- Myths about Water Fasting and Autophagy

- Water Fasting; its types, benefits, and how to harness it for all its benefits

- How to ease into fasting, doing it the right and easy way, and understanding your routine

Everyone needs autophagy in their lives, and no one benefits from being overweight; rather, being overweight poses some health risks. Being overweight can cause inflammation, heart-related diseases as well as others.

Can you imagine how active and alive you will feel after losing some weight within a few weeks into autophagy? Furthermore, imagine how happy your friends and family will be when they see you radiating with more energy than ever before? All these benefits can be achieved with less stress and without starving yourself to death.

Autophagy and water fasting are the best choices for those who wish to have a healthy and clean body.

Chapter 1: Autophagy/Water Fasting

Over time, the metabolic activities in a healthy human body lead to cellular damage. Sadly, the rate at which our cells are damaged increases as we age due to stress, exposure to radiation among others. However, Autophagy can help the body remove such damaged cells as well as old cells that are no longer active but are still present in the body. If such cells are not removed, it may lead to inflammatory diseases as well as other harmful cardiovascular diseases.

Autophagy is derived from the combination of two Greek words which are: **auto** which means 'self' and **phagy** which means to 'engulf.' Therefore, autophagy means the engulfment of the body's cells or tissues as part of the normal metabolic processes which is both beneficial and protective.

Over the years, fasting has been used as a way of shedding weight.

The fast diet also known as water fasting or water cleanse, involves the consumption of water alone over a specific period, with no calories intake at all for a set period. This fast is in stark contrast with caloric restriction in which the daily consumption is cut down to about 20 to 40%.

What you eat during a water fast?

When doing a water fast, you can't by any means eat anything. Also, you are not expected to drink something else besides water. In water fasting, the average daily intake of water is about 2-3 liters.

This fast should last for at least 24 hours, and 72 hours at most. Water fasting beyond this period requires guidance and supervision by medical professionals because some health risks might come with it. It is typical of water fast to make you feel weak and dizzy. However, try not to get involved in any overwhelming physical work. Also, stay away from long-distance driving to avoid an accident.

NB:

- *In water fasting, everything is forbidden except water, and it usually lasts for 24-72 hours.*

- *Do not exceed* this period without proper medical monitoring.

In recent times, this method of fasting has become more popular as an effective way of shedding weight.

Some of the reasons why people go on a water fast:

- For religious purpose

- For weight loss

- For detoxification

- For its associated health benefits

- For those preparing for a medical treatment

However, most people go on water fasting primarily because of its associated health benefits.

The Origin of Autophagy

Early in the 1950s, Christian de Duve a Belgian scientist discovered the process of autophagy by accident while working on insulin.

Between 1970 and 1980, researchers began taking a closer look at the process of cellular autophagy. At that time, little information was available about the importance of autophagy. After so many years of hard work, a significant milestone was achieved in 1983, when Yoshinori Ohsumi, discovered genes responsible for the regulation of autophagy in yeast. From his discovery, he found out that autophagy was absent in yeast cells lacking those genes and such cells were unable to repair themselves. In 2016, he was awarded a Nobel Prize for this great discovery.[1][2]

The interesting thing about this discovery is how the cell responds to increased stress, nutrient deficiency, deprivation of energy and cellular injuries by increasing the rate of cellular autophagy but where the stress is eliminated, the process of autophagy goes back to the regular rate (maintenance mode).

With more desires to fully understand the process of autophagy, more research works are now aimed at understanding the relationship between aging and autophagy, and the effect of stress on this process.

There is a general theory that there is a relationship between aging and the rate of autophagy as well. According to evidence, the process that enhances autophagy will also help to extend the lifespan of such individual. Another research reported that cell related aging attributed to the accumulation of damaged cells without proper means of removal. Since autophagy helps to remove damaged cells thereby slowing down the process of aging, scientists are looking at ways of extending the life expectancy of humans by inducing autophagy.

Benefits of Fasting:

1. **It enhances the body's fitness.** Fasting helps the body to burn fats, and as such, the body will feel lighter and such individual can be said to be fit.

2. **Promotes greater satiety.** Your adipocytes produce various

hormones (acting as an endocrine organ), such as your leptin which regulates the way you feel. When you fast; however, you burn most of these stored fatty tissues, your leptin levels drop automatically (creating a leptin-deficient environment). Hence, whenever the little amount of leptin is produced, the effect is heightened, and your body becomes more responsive to leptin thereby modulating how you feel after a meal.

3. **Enhanced metabolism.** Leptin is also known as the (satiety hormone) also stimulate the production of thyroid hormones. Thus, enhanced leptin responsiveness will directly increase the rate of metabolism.

4. **Facilitates fat loss and ketosis.** Fat-loss or ketosis can be accomplished either by eating a Ketogenic Diet or by fasting. A Ketogenic Diet helps to burn out stored fat which is harmful rather than helpful to the body organs

such as the liver, the kidneys, and the blood vessels.

5. **Enhances insulin sensitivity:** When you fast, the body secretes a lesser amount of insulin which in turn increases insulin sensitivity.

6. **Boosts cardiovascular health:** Fasting is recommended for those who wish to improve their cardiovascular function and have normal blood pressure.

7. **Reduced blood pressure.** Most people experience lower BP while fasting. This effect could be as a result of lower salt consumption and increased salt loss through urine.

8. **Lower blood sugar.** The blood sugar could drop as much as over 30 percent within a few days of fasting, and if care is not taken, the person could become hyperglycemic.

9. **Decreases blood triglycerides.** The triglycerides content of the

blood drops low while an individual is fasting which helps to increase the blood flow within the blood vessels which could have been narrowed by fat components.

10. **Better heart condition.** Fasting has been found to help reduce the accumulation of free radicals within the body. Free radicals are harmful to the muscles of the heart.

11. **Could slow the rate of aging and prolong your lifespan.** There have been positive results obtained from animal studies to prove that fasting could prolong lifespan. Also, when the blood is cleaned regularly, it slows down the process of aging and improves the health of an individual.

12. **Suppresses inflammation.** Although several factors cause inflammation, an unhealthy diet could lead to increased production of free radicals which in turn could cause inflammation. Food items such as alcohol, refined food items,

fried foods, etc. are all sources of free radicals.

13. **Reduces the effects of Oxidative Stress.** When the rate at which free radicals are produced is higher than the rate at which it is eliminated, it accumulates in the body thereby causing oxidative stress which is damaging to the cells of the body.

14. **Enhances cellular recycling process.** Senescent cells accumulate in our body as we age. But when we fast, the body activates the process of self-digestion, and along the line, malignant cells are also destroyed.

15. **Growth regulation.** It has been found that insulin-like growth factor 1 (IGF-1) could lead to the proliferation of cancer. But fasting suppresses the production of IGF-1.

16. **Protects the brain.** Research works carried out on the function of the brain and aging have

revealed one could age gracefully by fasting regularly.

17. **Promotes a healthy stress response.** Moderate stress is beneficial to the brain especially when it is infrequent, and fasting can induce such stress. Moderate stress triggers a series of activities that are protective to the brain cells (neurons).

18. **Promotes recovery from an injury.** Though the mechanism is not fully understood, research from animal models has shown that intermittent fasting helps the healing process.

19. **Supports healthier skin collagen production.** Your skin is a reflection of your diet. Accumulation of glucose can compromise the structure of the collagen, but fasting can help you overcome this challenge and give your skin that glow.

Side Effects of Fasting

Everyone fasts for various reasons such as: to lose weight, for a religious purpose, for healthy living and the list goes on. A fast could either be mild or strict (ranging from liquid only such as juice, tea, coffee and the likes to no food, no fluid). Although fasting comes with a lot of benefits, it also has its associated downsides which could either be short term or long term. These effects vary from one individual to another.

Poor weight management. Many people tend to crave for and consume more calories after a long period of fasting which will inevitably counteract all the progress made by fasting.

Short-term downsides. Fasting could have several adverse effects such: dizziness, headaches, outbursts, weakness, low blood pressure, gouts/gall stones among others.

Long-Term downsides. Continuous prolonged fasting could weaken the immune system and affect vital organs such as the kidneys and the liver. When an individual abstains from food over a long period, he becomes malnourished and could lead to an untimely death after the entire energy store of the body has been exhausted.

Dry Fast. Dry fasting is the most dangerous form of fasting in which an individual abstains from food and fluids. It could even lead to death if other underlying factors such as exertions, heat and the likes set in.

Water Fasting. There is a high tendency of losing the wrong type of weight while performing this form of fasting. This is because this form of fasting only allows the intake of water but restrict one from taking in calories. Although an individual could lose up to 0.9kg (2 pounds) 24-72 hours of water fasting, sadly, such weight loss can be a loss of carbohydrates, muscle mass and even water.

Possible dehydration. As funny as it may sound, water fasting could still cause dehydration because about 20-30 percent of our daily water intake comes from the food we eat. Thus, if we consume the same amount of water as we do on average days, we could experience some symptoms of dehydration such as light-headedness, dizziness, constipation, headaches, weakness, nausea, etc. To prevent such unwanted side effects, you may need to increase your water consumption.

Possibility of experiencing Orthostatic Hypotension. This type of hypotension is usually common among those whose fast. You might have experienced something similar when you get up suddenly, and then you feel dizzy or lightheaded. That feeling is caused by a sudden drop in the blood pressure, and such ones are prone to fainting. If you think you are experiencing orthostatic hypotension, then it means your body is not compatible with water fasting.

Water fasting could worsen a medical condition: Those with certain medical conditions should avoid water fasting as it could worsen such conditions:

- **Gout**: Gout is caused by an accumulation of Uric acid in the joints, and water fasting could increase its production.

- **Diabetes**: In Type I and type II diabetes, fasting could aggravate the side effect of diabetes.

- **Chronic kidney disease**: Those with chronic kidney condition should avoid water fast as it may worsen such condition.

- **Eating disorders**: Bulimia nervosa could be enhanced by fasting. There is more than sufficient evidence to back this up.

- **Heartburn:** Heartburn may be induced by fasting as the body will keep producing gastric acid which helps the digestion process.

Precautions to Take When Fasting

Fasting has a lot of advantages. However, fasting is not meant for everyone. To better understand the theory of fasting, let us compare Fasting to a tool (such as an arrow) which can either be used properly or misused. Holding to that, we will use the archery metaphor to explain the effective use and the misuse of fasting/autophagy. A hunter could have different sizes and tips of arrows in his quiver. When he finds an antelope, he will use a sharp wooden arrow, but when faced by a lion or bear, he would go for something stronger: probably an arrow with metallic tips. The point is don't use the wrong method for the right purpose.

Who should avoid fasting

Pregnant and breastfeeding mothers. Whether you have a child you're breastfeeding or one who is still in your uterus, you need all the calories you can get; both the mother and the infant need to be fed well to stay nourished and healthy.

Underaged students and those below 18 should avoid Fasting. Children under the age of 18 are still growing and need all the vital nutrients and minerals to have healthy growth and development.

Those that are underweight and/or malnourished. If you find it difficult to tell whether you are malnourished or not, you could ask your physician or a trusted friend. Those having an eating disorder such as bulimia are included in this category.

Individuals who have Type-2 Diabetes. Fasting has been used over the years as a means of reversing the effect of Type-2 diabetes.

However, you still need to consult your physician before beginning a fast.

Who needs to be cautious?

Another group of individuals who also need to be cautious is those with occasional gastroesophageal reflux disease (GERD). Those who fall into this category need to check with their physician as well if they wish to fast and must be closely monitored.

There are solid pieces of evidence to prove that GERD could be aggravated by fasting and the symptoms could become worsened. This possible worsening is because during fasting, the stomach will be devoid of food and there will be nothing which the gastric juice would digest.

Individuals on medications need to be cautious while fasting as the fasting periods could overlap when such drugs would be taken especially those medications that would require you to eat before using them.

In addition, those on cancer therapy and other medical treatment must be cautious and should have an in-depth discussion with their physician before fasting.

Chapter 2: How Does Autophagy Work?

Forms of Autophagy

First, let us identify the three types of autophagy.[3] They are:

- **macroautophagy**
- **microautophagy**
- **chaperone-mediated autophagy**

All the three forms of autophagy involve the process of breaking down and reproducing certain specific components found within the lysosome.

Macro-autophagy: During this process, all waste materials within a cell are transported via a double membrane-bound vesicle, (an autophagosome).[4] The waste can then fuse with the cytoplasmic lysosome (forming an autolysosome).

Micro-autophagy: This is in sharp contrast with the process of macro-autophagy. In this case, the cellular wastes to be digested are not transported via a membrane, but rather, they are mopped up by the cytoplasmic lysosome itself (via the membrane). And through this process, the cell cleans itself.[5]

NB: During the process of both macro-autophagy & microautophagy, both selective and non-selective processes can be employed when the cell wants to transport large molecules to be recycled or cleaned up.

Chaperone-mediated autophagy: During this process, the cell utilizes chaperone proteins (such as Hsc-70) which are found on the surface of the lysosomal membrane. These chaperones can then bind to the desired protein thereby facilitating their movement across the selectively permeable membrane.[6]

From a molecular point of view, the entire process of autophagy could be divided into five stages which are:

- Initiation

- Elongation

- Autophagosome formation

- Fusion

- Autolysosome formation

- Degradation

In summary, cellular components to be degraded are collected together to form a macro/large molecule which is then broken down into smaller/micro molecules such as fatty acids, amino acids, glucose, and nucleotides.

Thus, such micro molecules will be available for use by the cell to form larger molecules. This process helps to renew the cells and therefore produce healthy cells.

Cell death occurs to ensure a balance between good and healthy cells and those that are senescent.

Autophagy is a survival mechanism that is imperative to the survival of cells especially when subjected to stressful conditions such as nutrient deprivation. Also, it helps the cell eliminate toxic materials, like pathogens, infections, and damaged organelles.

Autophagy Vs. Apoptosis

Apoptosis is defined as the programmed death of a cell which occurs as part of the cell's normal activities.

But one may wonder how apoptosis is related to autophagy. Scientists believe that autophagy is a highly selective process by which a particular organelle(s) are eliminated from a cell. Also, there is tangible evidence to prove that one process does not control the other. However, there are reasons to believe that autophagy as a whole is a process of cell death that is independent of apoptosis.

Researchers are particularly interested in the association between autophagy and apoptosis because they believe that such knowledge could aid the treatment of cancer and management of neurodegenerative diseases such as Alzheimer's disease based on the capacity of both processes to regulate cell death. When such knowledge is available, autophagy could then be used as a therapeutic tool to eliminate harmful cells while protecting the healthy ones[7]

How to Induce Autophagy

Fossil evidence from the past showed strong and healthy bones and teeth of humans at an early age of our history, yet there are also evidences to show that most humans from ancient history went for days without food.

Some reasons responsible for this include:

- **They had to work to eat:** The early men had to farm or hunt before they could eat unlike today when you can easily stroll to a grocery store to buy foodstuffs.
- **They felt weak regularly:** Lack of energy is one of the primary triggers of autophagy

Here is a simple comparison between the ancient food environment and the modern food environment:

- **Most people have access to food:** Today, there is more than enough food for everyone to eat. Food is affordable and easily accessible to all.
- **People no longer have to work hard to eat:** Most of us drive down to the

grocery or talk a short stroll down to the store with money in our pocket and VOOM, we can purchase high caloric food with a little amount of money. As a matter of fact, high caloric food items are the cheapest items on the shelf. We no longer have to farm or hunt before eating.

- **We can eat anytime we want:** If one is not cautious, you might find yourself munching one thing or another for most of the day.

In our modern-day society, an average individual can't go a day without taking in food substances that are capable of inducing autophagy. However, we do not engage in sufficient rigorous activities that could help expend energy to be energy deficient. In simple terms, our input is not equivalent to our output (i.e., what we take in does not equate what goes out). This is in sharp contrast with the eating environment in which our ancestors lived, and if they were given similar opportunity today, they would fall over each other to have a fill. In our modern society, the most important thing we need to focus on is finding ways to activate the process of autophagy.

Autophagy occurs in virtually all the cells in our body. However, this activity is further enhanced in response to stressful activities such as hunger, and starvation. Additional activities that could be considered as adequate stressors include exercise, fasting. Research has shown that both activities have helped to prevent age-related diseases, induce weight loss, and can extend the life-span of an individual.

Four ways of inducing autophagy while carrying out your normal daily activities:

1. Fasting. Due to our hectic lifestyles, it is good to know that you can still control your eating habits and your lifestyle. One of the good triggers of autophagy isn't very hard to imagine at all. One of the more popular triggers you can practice is intermittent fasting (IMF), and you can still take other liquids such as water and tea/coffee.

What is intermittent fasting? This is a form of time-restricted fasting in which an individual abstains from food for a specified period. We have different types of intermittent fasting such as the eating window and alternate-day fasting.

How long before autophagy is triggered? Well, studies have shown that fasting for 1-2 days (24-

48 hours) usually produces the best effect.[8] However, this is an impossible task for most people. Still, many people can still fast for half a day (12 hours) or more without too much trouble, and this can be done by eating once or twice daily. For instance, if you had your last meal by 7 PM today, the next meal should come by 7 AM or thereabout. That way, you would have fasted for 12 hours. You could then have the next meal by 7 PM.

Another option is to have your regular meal at regular intervals then you go on a two to three day (2-3 days) fast. When it comes to alternate fasting, you could decide to cut down on your calorie intake during the fasting periods by eating only 1-2 meals (≤ 500 calories) then you can have your fill of calories on regular days.

Autophagy Fasting

Our bodies see any form of fasting as stress, and this sounds logical when you give it a bit of thought. During a fasting period, you feel hungry, and your body will attempt to maximize the distribution of your energy.

Below are the different kinds of fasts you can pick.

- **Long Fasts.** These type of fasts require you to stay away from any form of eating for a minimum of 24 hours.

- **Dry Fast.** This is a brutal form of fasting which remains popular despite its harshness. It is a hazardous form of fasting where you can't eat or drink anything. It is not advisable to stay away from drinking water; therefore, I would advise you to stay away from this type of fast for your health's sake.

- **Water Fast.** Water Fasting is another popular fasting type (and the reason for this book). This form of fasting is known for its autophagous, weight loss, detox, and anti-aging benefits. It requires you to stay away from eating but recommends you drink water or other forms of liquid depending on the variation of water fasting you are attempting. However, drinks such as protein shakes or juice are a "No" for it because they contain calories that could lead you to retain your weight.

Long fasts can enhance autophagy and weight loss. The loss of function by a stem cell can be reversed by one 24-hour fast, significantly improving their regeneration abilities.

You are probably thinking how long it will take you to fast to induce autophagy. Different research has shown that a fasting period of 24 to 36 hours would induce autophagy, suggesting that intermittent water fasting is another good option, although not as reliable as long water fasts, although

Fasting is about staying away from calories, to enable your body to reset its metabolic activities. This, however, doesn't mean you stay away from drinking water or specific teas, provided you don't add sugars, or you're selective about the natural sweeteners you add.

2. Ketogenic diets. Ketogenic diets (KD) are food substances that are very rich in fat but low in carbohydrates. Taking KD produces similar effects as fasting. KD comprises more than 75% of your daily fat consumption and less than 5-10% of calories obtained your daily carb consumption. When this is consumed, it triggers the body to undergo the process of gluconeogenesis (a process in which the body derives energy from non-carbohydrate sources such as fat).

Some food suggestions for KD includes eggs, avocado, fermented cheeses, seeds, nuts, butter, olive oil, fish, vegetables, vitamins, etc.

Ketone bodies are produced in response to KD which has several protective advantages. Multiple research works have shown that autophagy induced by starvation has neuro-protective advantages. For instance, the result of a study showed that rats fed with KD diets experienced a lesser amount of brain injury during a seizure.

3. Exercise. Exercise is one of the best stressors that are capable of triggering autophagy. One good thing about exercise according to reports from scientists is that it can trigger autophagy in many organs at the same time such as the liver, the muscles, the pancreas, the adipocytes, etc.[9]

Exercise helps the body regenerate and produce new tissues by breaking down worn out tissues and stimulating the body to create new ones. However, the amount of activity needed to stimulate autophagy is not yet clearly defined. For instance, 30 mins of exercise is enough to trigger autophagy in cardiac and skeletal muscles.

4. Sleep

Even though a vast majority of people replace rest time with binge-watching television, doing more work, and hanging out with friends, our body works at it's optimum when we acknowledge it's circadian rhythm or natural biological clock. This clock is in control of our sleeping cycles, as well as controls the process of autophagy.

It is vital to respect our circadian rhythm because it controls metabolic activities in the body. During our sleep, hormones are produced and released in our bodies. The absence of rest and sleep is seen as a stressful and distressing activity, and it negatively affects our health.

Sleep is therefore crucial in inducing autophagy as an absence of it alters the process of autophagy, and significantly slows it down.

Water-Fasting, Autophagy, and Anti-Aging – The Intersection

Aging is a result of a decrease in the rate and amount of autophagy, leading to accumulation of higher amounts of junks and cellular damage.

As organisms age, they experience a decrease in their autophagous capacities which means that they cannot service and repair themselves as they used to any longer. As a result of this, there'll be an accumulation of cell damage, and after some time (days or months or years), most of the cells become damaged or malfunctioning, losing their ability to function at an optimal level. If this degradation gets to vital organs, death becomes inevitably close.

Autophagy occurs in a cycle, fluctuating at different rates at different times of the day. An increased level of eating reduces autophagy, while fasting increases it.

Therefore, if the result of aging is a decreased rate of autophagy and an increase in damage accumulation, and the effect of fasting is an increased rate of autophagy, then fasting combats aging.

Anti-aging is the greatest significant benefit that comes with water fasting. Water fasting is, in fact, the most effective anti-aging strategy available. Therefore, anything that enhances autophagy can have anti-aging effects.

We won't enter a fasting state if we eat food every time, and will in principle, never speed up autophagy.

Remember, eating constantly, or "grazing" is a pro-aging activity, so, don't eat all the time.

Chapter 3: Myths and Symptoms of Water Fasting and Autophagy

Common Myths About Autophagy

There are lots of unknown facts about Autophagy – how it is measured, the mechanism of action, whether it is beneficial or not, and the effective quantity. There are also a lot of superstition and fabrications concerning autophagy.[10]

To begin Autophagy, you must fast for 3 to 5 days

To initiate autophagy, you must stimulate energy depletion and use up the body's own energy.

A person that eats a standard diet without cutting our protein or carbohydrates would have to fast for a minimum of 3 days to enter a ketotic state and initiate autophagy. Consequently, autophagy is controlled by maintaining stability between AMPK (or the AMP-activated protein kinase) and mTOR (or the mechanistic target of rapamycin).

You can certainly speed up the initiation of autophagy if you begin with lower energy stores, that is, you limit carbs and avoid overeating protein.

If your diet is based on whole foods, you are expected to enter the zone of therapy faster because there is a minimal quantity of excess energy in your body.

A 24-Hour Fast will give you Autophagy

Unfortunately, boosting autophagy is difficult when on a one-day fast unless you are doing lots of exercises while fasting.

Don't limit yourself to naïve the belief that you will enter autophagy if you fast for 16 hours because that is not a long enough timeframe. Some of the reasons why are:

- You must digest the nutrients from your last meal, so fasting is not initiated instantly
- After the absorption of nutrients, metabolism continues for four more hours after your food was eaten
- Foods like vegetables, fat, fiber and protein have a longer period of digestion.

You get into the state of fasting after 5 or 6 hours without eating because before this period, there is still food in your system, and you are using up calories from the previous food.

If your last meal was by 7 pm, your actual physiological fast does not start till midnight. So, if you are on a 16 or 20 hour fast, you have only spent 12 hours in a fasting state, which is not enough to initiate autophagy.

In addition to other hormonal advantages, Other benefits you would get are lowered inflammatory processes, reduced insulin. The appropriate period is 24 hours or more, as you would want to remain in the therapeutic zone for more than 2 hours.

More Autophagy is helpful

It would be beneficial to fast for at least 3 days to achieve meaningful autophagy. This will fight against tumors and malignancies and energize stem cells. Although, increased autophagy does not necessarily mean it would be helpful.

The harmful effects of excessive autophagy include:

- Excess autophagy might result in sarcopenia and muscle atrophy, which would, in turn, shorten your lifespan
- It makes tumor cells resistant to environmental stressors, making it harder for them to be killed.
- Autophagy promotes the replication of bacteria such as Brucella.
- ATG6/BECN1 which is the crucial gene for autophagy is a tumor suppressor. Although, in some cases, it might allow cancer to thrive by feeding it.

Although autophagy is incredible and it can help to improve your health, it is not always ideal. You would not want to always be in a state of autophagy throughout your life because there might be some side-effects that have not yet been discovered.

The best option is to alternate between autophagy and fasting- to practice extended fasts but not turn it into a do-or-die affair. We would not want to turn autophagy into a new diet ritual, right?

Starving is the same as Autophagy

From all that we have discussed, autophagy is not the same as starvation. You might think that fasting and going without food causes starvation, but that is a wrong approach to it.

Fasting results in starvation because you are not getting calories from food. Although, it would be almost impossible for the energy stores in your body to be completely depleted. These are the reasons:

- Autophagy degrades worn-out cells and proteins that will serve as an energy source again; when energy is insufficient, the body has no choice but to rechannel the less significant processes that won't take place when eating.

- You go into a ketotic state after fasting for several days. In a ketotic state, the main source of energy for the muscles and brain is ketones and fat. This alters everything because you would have to start using your biggest energy reserve- the adipose tissue. A car that uses up fuel after 100 miles might become starved, but a truck that has fuel stored in thousands of gallons can keep running for thousands of miles without hitting starvation. Remember, fat is the body's primary source of fuel.

- Everybody has at least some body fat. Body fat is a reservoir of energy that the body can survive on. People with as low as 10% of body fat have between 40 to 50,000 calories in "reserve." That is enough for weeks, even months.

- Simple autophagy lengthens lifespan and endurance. It is the primary cause of a longer life as observed in the restriction of calories.

In my point of view, autophagy and fasting are not the same as your body experiences the process of self-rejuvenation and restoration which does not happen when you eat. You might think it is starvation, but this is not correct. Even if you want to think of it as starvation, a small amount won't hurt; in fact, it is very beneficial to your health.

Autophagy develops your muscles

Developing your muscles without additional fuel or by going without food is extremely difficult because you need calories to build muscles.

Muscle development also requires the initiation of protein synthesis, which can only be done by eating protein. Fasting means that food is not the source of protein for your body, so your body is in a state of catabolism- break down, instead of anabolism- building up.

Hypothetically, autophagy also causes the degradation of worn-out proteins that are wandering about in your cells, and they are converted to synthesize proteins, but you still lack some specific amino acids such as leucine that are needed for protein synthesis in the muscle.

In a few cases, an overweight person that recently started resistance workouts may develop muscle while simultaneously losing fat. Although, it is mainly stimulated by the recent strength training.

Autophagy consumes flabby skin

It is believed that autophagy can consume excess skin that might be obvious after a recent weight loss and make it tighter. Although, there are some exceptions to this.

- Research conducted in 2014 in Japan discovered that old fibroblasts had reduced autophagy. Fibroblasts produce collagen in the skin, the cause of wrinkles and flabby skin.
- Another research conducted in Korea in 2018 discovered that old fibroblast has a higher rate of generating waste that then causes aging of the skin. The researchers concluded that autophagy is

essential for reversing the process of aging by maintaining the health of the fibroblast.

Autophagy might help to reduce the rate at which the skin ages, but in reality, it does not consume flabby skin. It just promotes the processes that are responsible for the skin's elasticity and tightness.

In situations of excessive weight loss, autophagy and fasting can help to avoid excess flabby skin. You would certainly have some flabby skin after you have lost a lot of weight. Although, if your weight loss were achieved through fasting, there would be increased autophagy which would enable your skin to adjust to the new weight quickly.

Diets involving caloric restrictions in the absence of autophagy might generate a larger amount of flabby skin. Various studies have discovered that autophagy is vital to the functioning of the fibroblast and production of collagen.

Autophagy is not inhibited by fat

Though fat does not boost the levels of insulin as much as proteins or carbs, it would still make you feel full.

A ketotic state enhances macroautophagy of the brain through the activation of Sirt1 (also known as NAD-dependent deacetylase sirtuin-1). Ketone bodies promote intermediate autophagy that is aimed at some substrates and amino acids. Production of ketone bodies, including beta-hydroxybutyrate is increased during starvation and fasting, and they are also increased while on a ketogenic diet.

Although, mTOR reacts to all calories and not just glucose and amino acids. Additional energy from any source prevents autophagy.

Autophagy might not be completely inhibited by fat; it will reduce it to an extent. The quantity of fat that you consume determines if autophagy would be inhibited by fat. Small quantities of fat such as one tablespoon of MCT oil (concentrated medium chain fatty acids derived from coconut oil) might enhance intermediate autophagy due to an increase in the number of ketone bodies. Though, it is excessive once it exceeds 100 calories.

Autophagy is not inhibited by BCAAs

Amino acids are the major constituents of Branched-Chain Amino Acids, and it would certainly inhibit autophagy regardless of the quantity.

If you are in a ketotic state during your fast, and autophagy is stable, you should not be worried about muscle loss. Due to the increased ketone bodies, they both antagonize muscle catabolism.

Muscle is only lost if you move out of ketosis and quit autophagy without continuing with adequate protein and nutrients. The funny thing is that consuming BCAAs might result in that by tilting you towards a fed state and stopping ketosis.

Although it is not required, consuming BCAAs while fasting isn't so bad since you are using up glucose, hence, there is an increase in the level of blood glucose.

Consuming meat prevents autophagy

People believe that consuming meat or being on a protein-rich diet inhibits autophagy throughout your lifetime and speeds up the process of aging.

The essential factor in autophagy is the number of times you eat. It doesn't matter if you limit your meat and protein, once you eat three times in one day and do not fast for more than 24 hours, you might still not gain any relevant autophagy.

Additionally, autophagy is inhibited by insulin and carbohydrates so a vegan diet that is entirely based on plants would not cause autophagy too if you are eating too often.

Autophagy is not interrupted by fruits

The liver metabolizes fructose present in fruits and stores it as glycogen. Extra fructose is quickly changed into triglycerides. Autophagy is interrupted by fruits, and ketosis is stopped because it replenishes glycogen stores in the liver. Liver glycogen determines the balance between AMPK and mTOR. The liver acts as the primary center for energy metabolism and nutrient condition.

If you are eating only fruit with little or no fat or protein, you might remain in a state of catabolism, but it is not the same as autophagy. Autophagy is different from catabolism and loss of muscle. It is possible to be in extreme autophagy, and all your muscles are intact if you are in more extreme ketotic state and it is possible to lose a lot of muscle in the absence of autophagy.

Fruit is acceptable, and it is healthy in certain quantities. Although, it is not an ideal food that retains you in an autophagy every time.

Autophagy is inhibited by coffee

Autophagy is not inhibited by drinking coffee; neither will it break your fast. In reality, coffee enhances ketosis and autophagy.

Polyphenols present in coffee will promote autophagy on its own, though it is also enhanced by the drink via other methods. Caffeine stimulates lipolysis- the using up of fatty acids, this reduces insulin levels, enhances ketone bodies and increases AMPK

Black Coffee without cream, milk or sweeteners; which might increase insulin and inhibit the fast, promotes autophagy. Dairy and milk increase IGF-1 too that in turn makes mTOR active. Sweeteners with zero calorie increase insulin through the cephalic phase response that promotes insulin inside the gut.

It is risky to include MCT oil to your coffee; make sure it does not exceed one tablespoon.

It is impossible for autophagy to occur while eating

The truth is that the most efficient and certain way to start autophagy is to go without food and fast. Although there are some foods that enhance autophagy

They include

- Ginger which induces autophagy

- Medicinal mushroom induces autophagy

- Sulforaphane in cruciferous vegetables and broccoli speeds up autophagy

- Polyphenols from vegetables and dark berries induce autophagy

- Turmeric and Curcumin speeds up autophagy

- Resveratrol in grape skin, red wine, and dark berries speeds up autophagy

The precaution is that you might still need to limit your caloric intake mildly and you won't achieve the total benefits of autophagy.

These are only a few examples of some calorie containing foods that can enhance the process of autophagy

Autophagy is inhibited by exercise

Exercise is a great way to speed up autophagy. It initiates autophagy in the brain and peripheral tissues. Resistance workouts speed up mTOR signaling. Although not in the same manner as eating. Exercise only causes translocation of the mTOR complex nearer to the cell membrane and readies it for activation as soon as eating commences. Exercising implies that there is an increased sensitivity to mTOR activation, and it results in additional growth after work-out.

Also, long-term resistance workouts turn on autophagy and lower muscle apoptosis by regulating IGF-1 and its receptors.

After fasting, exercising is the closest activity that speeds up autophagy and enhances overall wellbeing. The most effective way is to do both and do them regularly.

Common Myths About Fasting

Next, this part disproves the common fallacies about snacking, the frequency of meals and fasting.

You will gain weight if you do not eat breakfast

The most important of the day is breakfast. There is a widespread misconception that there is something unique concerning breakfast.

Most people think that missing breakfast results in weight gain, cravings, and extreme hunger.

Though a lot of observational studies have discovered connections between not eating breakfast and obesity, this is because the person that typically skips breakfast is not very health conscious.

Although there might be some individual differences, it doesn't matter whether you eat breakfast.

However, kids who eat the first meal of the day have been found to be better at schoolwork. A few people have also achieved success with long-term weight loss indicating that they eat breakfast most times. This is one of those individual differences. For a few people, breakfast might be helpful while for others, it might not be.

Eating increases your metabolic rate

Consume a lot of small meals to continue the metabolic process. A lot of people think that eating additional meals results in higher metabolism, so your body depletes calories. The truth is, during the process of digestion and absorption of food, the body uses a particular quantity of energy. This is known as TEF(the thermic effect of food), and it is proportional to 0-3% fat, 5-10% carbs, and 20-30% protein.[11]

Usually, TEF is about 10% of the total quantity of consumed calories. Although, the important thing is not the frequency of your meals, but the number of calories consumed.

Consuming six meals with a calorie content of 600 gives the same benefit as eating three meals with a calorie content of 1,000. In the two instances, the average thermic effect, which is 10% is 300 calories. This is evidenced by much feeding research in humans that have discovered that reducing or increasing the number of times you eat does not affect the calories used.[12]

Hunger is decreased by frequent eating

A few people think that snaking stops extreme hunger and cravings. However, a lot of research has studied this, and the outcomes are mixed. Though some research hypothesizes that frequent eating results in decreased hunger.

Further research discovered no benefits and some determined, elevated levels of hunger.[1314]

One research compared six meals rich in protein to three other meals rich in protein, and it was discovered that the three meals were more effective for decreasing hunger.[15]

However, this is determined on an individual basis. If you experience a few cravings when you snack, you tend to binge-eat less; this might be a good idea.

There is no proof that eating or snacking decreases hunger for everybody.

Weight loss can be achieved with a lot of small meals

Eating frequent meals does not speed up the metabolic rate. It also does not decrease hunger.

If eating more meals does not affect the energy levels, then weight loss should not be affected. Science supports this. Most researches on this have discovered that the number of times you eat does not affect weight loss.[16]

For instance, research on 16 obese men and women did not discover any variation in appetite, weight, and loss of fat when contrasting three and six meals each day.[17]

Although if you discover that frequently eating makes it less hard to eat a few junk food and calories, maybe this would be beneficial to you.

For me, it is very stressful to eat frequently making it difficult to adhere to one healthy diet plan although it might be effective for some people.

The brain requires a steady supply of glucose

A few people think that if we do not consume carbs intermittently, our brain would be less active. The foundation of this is that the brain exclusively utilizes glucose as a source of energy. Although, what we often exclude is that the brain can effectively generate the glucose it requires via gluconeogenesis.

In a lot of cases, this might not be required because the body has a glycogen reservoir that can still supply the brain for a lot of hours.

While on a long-term fast, very low-carb diet or starvation can generate ketone bodies from dietary fats.

Ketone bodies generate energy for some of the brain decreasing the glucose needs greatly.

Thus, while on a long-term fast, the brain can still be sustained by consuming ketone bodies and glucose generated from fats and protein. From the history of evolution, it is pointless to think that we would not be able to live in the absence of a steady source of carbohydrates. If this were truly the case, then humans would have gone into extinction since.

Although a few people say that they experience hypoglycemia after going without food. If this happens to you, you should probably adhere to eating more meals, or confirm from your doctor before you make changes.

It is healthy to snack and eat frequently

The body cannot naturally remain in a fed state. During human evolution, we had to bear times of food shortages. This is proof that fasting for a short period initiates a process of cell repair known as autophagy where the cells utilize workout and malfunctioning proteins as a source of fuel. Autophagy can prevent aging and diseases such as Alzheimer's disease; it may even decrease the risk of cancer. Fasting at various times is very beneficial to metabolism.[18]

Also, some researchers have proposed that snacking and frequent eating can otherwise affect your health and increase the risk of diseases.

For instance, one research discovered that a diet that involves frequent eating and high amounts of calories could increase the risk of a fatty liver.[19]

Some observational studies have also discovered that people that eat frequently have an increased risk of colorectal cancer.[20]

Fasting makes your body go into starvation

The general thoughts concerning fasting at intervals are that it might tilt your body into a period of starvation, basically called adaptive thermogenesis. This can result in burning up fewer quantities of calories each day. Although this occurs with losing weight, irrespective of the strategy used. There is no proof that this is more common with intermittent fasting compared with other methods of weight loss.

There is proof that fasting for short-term increases metabolism. This is because of a sudden increase in noradrenaline (norepinephrine) which activates fat cells to degrade body fat and enhance the metabolic rate.

Research has discovered that fasting for about 48 hours can improve metabolic rate three times faster, although if you fast for a longer period, this can be modified, and the metabolic rate can be further reduced than the standard rate.

One research discovered that fasting at least once in 22 days did not result in a reduction in metabolism, but the subjects lost 4% of their body fat which is excellent for less than three weeks of fasting.[21]

There is a minimum amount of protein that can be utilized for every meal

Some people say that for every meal, only 30 grams of protein is digested and that we should eat meals every 2 or 3 hours to optimize muscle gain.

Although science does not back this up, research has shown that there is no obvious variation in muscle mass if you consume protein more frequently.[22] The overall quantity of protein consumed the most significant factor for most people, not the frequency of meals that contains protein.

You lose muscle when you undergo intermittent fasting

A few people think that fasting uses up muscles as an energy source.

Generally, this occurs when we diet, but there is no proof that this occurs with intermittent fasting compared to other strategies. Some researchers have proposed that intermittent fasting can effectively maintain muscle mass. Review research discovered that intermittent calorie limitation resulted in the same degree of weight loss seen in continuous calorie limitation but more decrease in muscle mass.[23]

Another research also involved the subject eating the same quantity of calories that they usually eat, with the exclusion of one large meal in the evening.[24]

The subjects lost body fat and had a fare increase (close to statistical significance) in their muscle mass, together with a lot of other benefits on the health.

A lot of bodybuilders also adopt intermittent fasting since it effectively maintains a large quantity of muscle with a reduced percentage of body fat.

It is unhealthy to carry out Intermittent Fasting

A few people assume that fasting might be hazardous, but this is nowhere close to the truth.

For instance, intermittent fasting alters the expression of genes that increase lifespan and prevent some diseases, and it has been discovered to increase the lifespan of tested animals. It is also very significant to metabolism, like enhanced sensitivity to insulin, and a decrease in different risk factors for heart diseases.

Also, it might be beneficial to mental health by increasing the levels of hormones known as BDNF (brain-derived neurotrophic factor). This may also prevent depression and other brain disorders.

You eat a lot while fasting intermittently

A few people say that intermittent fasting would not result in weight loss, because it makes you overeat. This might be true. People are likely to eat more food while fasting compared periods of not fasting. This means that they try to replace the calories that were lost while fasting by increased eating over the subsequent meals.

Although, this replacement is incomplete. A research discovered that people who went without food for an entire day ate an additional 500 calories the following day. So, they used up 2,400 calories on the days they fasted then replaced with 500 calories the following day. The overall decrease in calorie consumption was 1,900 calories which is quite a huge loss for just two days.[25]

Intermittent fasting lowers total food insulin and enhances metabolic rate. It lowers the levels of insulin, raises norepinephrine and enhances growth hormones in humans five times. As a result of these factors, intermittent fasting causes fat loss instead of gain. Review research conducted in 2014 discovered that fasting for 3-24 weeks resulted in a 4-7% reduction in stomach fat and weight loss of 3-8%. In this research, intermittent fasting resulted in a weight loss of 0.55 pound every week, compared to intermittent fasting that resulted in 1.65 pounds weight loss every week. In reality, intermittent fasting is the strongest strategy for weight loss worldwide. It is not at all true to say that it causes you to overeat and enter starvation mode and eventual weight gain.

Symptoms of Water Fasting

At the beginning of water fast you might notice a lot of beneficial effects and some side-effects. This is to be expected. We will be discussing these so that you can have a deeper knowledge of what your body is going through.

These symptoms are to be expected and should not cause any worry[26]

Hunger. This is caused by ghrelin secreted by the stomach as a reaction to an empty stomach or as an automatic secretion at the times when we usually feed. Do not be concerned; you won't die; neither are you starving; this is just a response to physiological hormones in your body.

Fatigue. This happens because the body has not fully adjusted to using ketones and fat as a source of energy.

Changes in mood. While the body is adjusting to the use of fat in place of sugar, the brain might be hypoglycemic at times, and this can cause brain haziness, depression, mental weakness, and irritability. You might feel headaches too.

Mental Weakness. We have adapted to our brain having a constant supply of sugar as an energy source; this low level of sugar generates less energy for the brain. Also, neurotransmitters are stimulated by the presence of food, so the levels decrease. If you are used to a ketogenic diet, you might not experience a lot of mental weakness on the first day.

Sleep Disturbances. For a few people, the fast makes them sleep peacefully while it is difficult for others. The more experienced you are with the ketogenic diet, the less hypoglycemia you will feel and you will observe a more peaceful sleep. It can be very beneficial to enhance your sleep with melatonin, adaptogenic spices such as ashwagandha, additional magnesium, and L-theanine as well.

Cravings. The brain responds to emotional feelings through cravings. Eating stimulates excitatory brain neurotransmitters like serotonin and dopamine. Generally, this is very good since eating is enjoyable. Fasting makes our brain too dependent on these feelings, and it causes an increase in the signals that would be sent to satisfy these feelings.

Rashes. You might probably experience rashes during your fast. Rashes happen in 10% of people, and the rashes are as a result of alterations in the skin microflora. Fasting reduces this microflora and a lot of harmful chemicals are released into the circulatory system and causes release Substance P and histamine in the skin that results in inflammation and rashes. They will fade eventually and are symptoms of a response to healing

Frequent urination. When the body degrades glycogen into energy, it also causes a release of water into the urinary system. Frequent urination is an expected response. You should also drink additional water than you normally drink and this will increase the quantity of your urine.

Tongue Changes. Your tongue might become black, white or yellow. This color change should be expected as part of the body's physiological detoxification.

Cold. When there is a sensation of food shortage by the body, the body starts to reduce the production of active thyroid hormone. This reduction helps to enhance the use of energy in the body, and the usual symptom is developing cold extremities and coldness all over the body.

When Should You Stop the Fast?

On the fourth day, you should have adapted, and it is simpler to continue the fast for longer if desired. Remember, some people who have disorders in metabolism or extreme stress might have some problems and might have to stop the fast early. These are the red flags you should look out for:

Excruciating Pain. If you experience excruciating pain while fasting, then stop the fast.

Increased loss of hair. Once you observe hair loss in chunks, stop the fast.

Extreme Hunger. You might experience a mild desire for food, but you should not feel actual hunger. If you feel this symptom, listen to your body and stop the fast.

Extreme Weight Loss. If you feel or look gaunt and tired, then stop the fast.

Loss of consciousness and fainting. If you experience loss of consciousness and faint, or you feel very dizzy, break the fast.

Palpitations. If you are experiencing heart palpitations that are making you worried or affecting your sleep, stop the fast.

Intense Vomiting or Diarrhea. This could result in the loss of excess electrolytes, and you should stop the fast.

You should not be embarrassed about breaking your fast early. The body becomes healthier and stronger after subsequent fasts. If you are experiencing major health issues, then you should engage in the water fast every 1-3 months, and eventually, you will experience a reduction in these stressful symptoms, and you would be able to fast for five whole days effortlessly.

Chapter 4: Starting a Water Fast

Common Kinds of Water Fasting:

Intermittent Water Fasting. There are distinct periods in each day for eating and fasting. This has an effect of limiting your daily eating window to predetermined hours, and it usually lasts for 8 to 24 hours.

Extended Fast. Extending your fast is a better way of burning body fat as it involves water fasting for a couple of days at a stretch. With prolonged fasting, the longer the fast, the more beneficial the process.

- 3-day water fast. You avoid eating food for 72 hours.

- 7 – 10-day water fast. The average time required to reach ketosis is roughly 72 hours. Therefore, you'll spend approximately 48 hours in ketosis

- 14 – 40-day water fast. In mental and physical terms, this is quite challenging. It is best suited for deeper healings.

Intermittent Fasting

Intermittent fasting (IF) is essentially an eating pattern whereby you alternate between periods of eating and fasting. Here, the time of eventual consumption of food is what is specified. The characteristics as mentioned above make it less of a diet and more of an eating pattern. Daily 16 hour fasts or fasting for 24 hours, twice a week are conventional intermittent fasting methods.

The act of fasting is one that has been evident in every stage of human evolution. For example, the hunter-gatherers of old did not have the means to preserve food as we do now neither was food available all year round. Since food was in short supply, humans evolved and gained the ability to live without food for extended periods.

As a matter of fact, intermittent fasting is a practice that is closer to our natural tendencies than eating 3 or more meals per day.

Intermittent fasting is usually used as a precursor to water fasting. It helps you ease into water fasting.

There are several intermittent fasting methods in existence, and they all have varying levels of effectiveness based on an individual's needs. Among the intermittent fasting methods, six methods are the most common. They are:

1. The 16/8 Method: Fast for 16 hours each day

When utilizing the method, you fast for 14 – 16 hours daily. This method restricts your eating window to 8-10 hours, during which you can have 2 or more meals. Popularized by fitness expert Martin Berkhan, the 16/8 method is also called the Leangains protocol.

The most common form of this method that produces the most success is by eating dinner and skipping breakfast the following day. In a scenario where your last meal was around 8 pm, and you don't eat until noon the following day, the fasting period is more or less 16 hours.

Women have been observed to perform better on slightly shorter fasts, so it is recommended that they fast for 14-15 hours. This method can be complicated initially for individuals that get hungry in the morning. Breakfast skippers, on the other hand, eat this way instinctively.

To help reduce hunger levels during the fast, you can drink coffee, non-caloric beverages, and water. Doing this helps with the transition to water fast.

In general, you should avoid junk foods or excessive amounts of calories during your eating window as eating such food items undermine the purpose of the fast. You should eat healthy foods.

2. **The 5:2 Diet: Fast for two days per week.**

This diet involves regularly eating for all but two days a week and is also referred to as the Fast Diet. On two selected days, calories consumed should be restricted to 500-600 calories on each day. For women, the recommended calorie intake is 500 calories while for men it's 600 calories. An example of this can involve eating normally on all days except Mondays and Thursdays, where you eat two small meals (300 calories per meal for men and 250 calories for women).

3. **Eat-Stop-Eat: Do a 24-hour fast, once or twice a week**

Here, a 24-hour fast is carried out once or twice a week. An example of this method is eating dinner on Monday at 7 pm and fasting until 7 pm the following day.

This method is not only limited to dinner to dinner cycles, but it can also be from breakfast one day to breakfast the following day and lunch to lunch. All cycles achieve the same result. Solid food is not allowed, but you can drink water, coffee, and non-caloric beverages.

You have to eat appropriately during eating periods while utilizing this method as a means of losing weight.

The downside to this method is the difficulty of a 24 hour fast for a lot of people. It is better to start from 14-16 hours fast and gradually work your way up to 24 hours fast.

4. **Alternate Day Fasting: Fast every other day.**

The alternate day fast is a full fast where you fast one day and eat the other day properly, i.e., you fast every other day. There are many variations of this method, and some of them have an allowance of 500 calories on fasting days.

Given the difficulty of a full fast every other day, I wouldn't recommend this variant for beginners.

This method is unpleasant and generally unsustainable in the long term because you will go to bed hungry several times in a given week.

5. The Warrior Diet: Fast during the day, eat a huge meal at night.

Here, you eat a small proportion of raw vegetables and fruits during the day. At night, you eat a substantial meal within a 4-hour eating window.

One of the first popular diets to incorporate intermittent fasting; the Warrior diet has similar food choices which are similar to a paleo diet-whole, unprocessed foods that are similar to the form in which they exist in nature.

Due to the large caloric intake involved, this isn't recommended during water fasting.

6. Spontaneous Meal Skipping: Skip meals when convenient.

Here, a strict intermittent fasting plan is not necessary for you to reap certain benefits of the fast. You can also skip meals when you are too busy to make a meal or when you are not hungry.

"People needing to eat every few hours to prevent themselves from losing muscle as a result of starvation" is a myth. Our bodies have what it takes to endure extended periods without food.

Using this method is as simple as skipping a meal if you are not hungry and eating healthy foods for subsequent meals. It can also involve carrying out a short fast while traveling. As long as you are skipping 1 or 2 meals, you are carrying out a spontaneous intermittent fast.

Extended Fasting

This can be embarked upon after about two weeks of intermittent fasting and/or ketogenic diet.

The three-day water fast

The three-day water fast is the most essential fast as three days is the period when your body's healing metabolism is unlocked. Three-day fasts also serve as stepping stones essential to moving on to longer fasts in which you undergo the deepest healing. Water fasting of any length can be made easier if you practice three-day fasts regularly.

At first, the three-day fast is the hardest of all fasts, and it is essential that you follow all the steps required for you to increase your chances of having a smooth experience.

Given its difficulty and excessive body demands, you must be comfortable with intermittent fasting before you can move on to the three-day fast.

As a beginner, the majority of the challenges of the three-day fast are physical because your body must learn to enter a state of ketosis.

So, let's look at what happens over these three days and their accompanying feelings.

Day 1: You will slowly deplete your carbohydrate reserves (glycogen) stored in your liver and the tissues surrounding your muscles on the first day. This won't be a challenge for you physiologically as you are familiar with the experience of surviving without food for a day. An extension of going without food for a day is going without food for three days, and this should enable you to focus on the physical changes occurring within you. Over these three days, you will often find yourself face to face with your ego in that you will face your addictions to food rather than giving in to the existential fear of survival presented by your ego.

Day 2: Your glycogen reserves will run out by the beginning of the second day. When you get to this point, your experience with fasting determines how you feel. Generally, you'll feel great because as your glycogen stores run out, your body will initiate ketosis. At this time, you will not suffer "loss of power."

Things will go differently if your body hasn't adapted to ketosis. In this scenario, after your glycogen reserves are depleted, your body will quickly search for an alternative energy source. Since your body hasn't learned to access the metabolic pathways that lead to the burning of fat through ketosis, it'll move to the closest source of energy: burning protein. The protein in question is your muscle tissue. However, you will not lose a significant portion of your muscle mass, probably just a few hundred grams, and this is until your body perfects ketosis usually by the end of the third day. At that point, any additional loss of muscle mass is negligible.

Around this time, you will feel weak, and this is a result of the relatively low levels of energy within you. As a result of burning through protein present in muscle tissue, you may experience aches in your back and leg muscles. The lack of energy and the low blood sugar levels contribute to the headaches you may experience during this period. The onset of detoxification can also contribute to this. You may feel dull aches around your kidneys as they work above their usual levels. This overwork is caused by the excessive amount of detoxification that the kidneys have to carry out to cope with the influx of toxins coming from the metabolism of proteins and fat cells. If you experience such symptoms, it's advisable to ensure you are getting enough fluids: at least a quart/liter or two per day. As there is no fixed minimal limit of the number of fluids you are required to drink, it becomes dependent on a person's level of toxicity. You should drink more if you have a high toxicity level. You should also reduce fluid intake if you have a low toxicity level. A lot of people can drink as much as 3-4 quarts/liters a day.

Be ready to feel awful while going through your initial three-day fasts. However, the "awful" feelings of general lack of energy and aches are very similar to what you experience when you have the flu and those times are usually bearable. You don't need to worry, neither do you need to give up at the point because you'll survive, and all these symptoms will pass.

Day 3: In terms of physiological processes, the third day is a continuation of the second day. In most cases, you feel at your worst at the end of the second day. You may also be at your lowest at the beginning of the third day. As the switch to ketosis approaches completion, things will begin to improve in terms of how you feel.

You'll probably be emotionally and physically drained after your first few three-day fasts. At the end of the third day, you don't need to do anything more as you would have accomplished your mission. After your first three-day fasts, you would have awakened your body's healing metabolism, and this will make subsequent fasts easier. Another thing you would have achieved is a significant degree of detoxification. Once your body has fully acclimatized to the three-day fast, you should take on a longer, more cleansing fast.

On getting to the end of the third day, you can reward yourself with freshly squeezed orange juice. As opposed to long fasts, there's no need for a long transition back to eating after the fast. It is important to note that the first few meals before and after the fast should be light: mostly fruits and vegetables. You shouldn't give in to your ego and eat too much. You should avoid this temptation and follow your healthy appetite. You would have undergone a few changes: your stomach would have shrunk, and your digestive system would have slowed down significantly. The direct result of this is that you need a few days to get things back to their optimum levels. If you honestly follow your appetite, you'll begin to eat normally in a few days.

The 7 – 10-day Water Fast

The best time to advance to this type of extended fast is when you are comfortable with the three-day fast, and your body can easily transit into a state of ketosis. You can only enjoy the full benefits of detoxification when your body begins to draw energy solely from your fat cells. The implication of this is a three-day fast is not enough to tackle the deeper issues that need healing.

The thought of undergoing a 7-10 day fast would be daunting especially if you struggled with your first few three-day fasts. Attending a fasting retreat is very helpful to gain the deepest experience from your fast.

7-10-day fasts are not as emotionally and physically demanding as you expect, and this is surely the case if you're healthy and don't have serious issues when you undergo detox. What makes the fast easier than it seems is because your body does the most difficult part of the work, which is the establishment of ketosis, during the first three days. The efficiency at which ketosis occurs increases significantly after the third day. The result of this increased efficiency is that you feel better overall and you have more energy at your disposal. As days progress, the fast feels like a celebration of the freedom you have gained over the daily need to eat food. A clearer consciousness usually accompanies this freedom, and a lighter body and these feel so good that a lot of people feel reluctant to go back to eating food after the fast. There's a significant degree of purity that comes with being able to live without the needs and addictions of food distracting you.

Let's take a look at how you will feel as you go through stages of 7-10-day water fast:

Days 1-3: The first three days of a 7-10 day fast are more or less the same as the entirety of a three day fast. As you gain experience, this part becomes easier and even enjoyable. Your body's ability to undergo ketosis will improve immensely over time.

Days 4-6: Your body will begin to heal and carry out detoxification once you fully enter ketosis. Certain symptoms will make you aware of the stage: your breath, general body odor, and even your sweat will begin to stink. This occurs because your body expels toxins through your skin. As a result of these physiological stages, you may want to avoid frequent social interactions. The upside to this is as you witness your body expelling such repulsive things, it makes you appreciate the fact that you have gotten rid of them. This also gives you the willpower to take up fasting again in the future; even it was hard for you in the beginning. To reap the full benefits, you should convert to water fasting on the fourth or fifth day of your first 7-10 day fast - especially when your tongue produces an unpleasant metallic tasting froth.

The detoxification can place a significant burden on the kidneys and muscles, causing them to ache. Fortunately, the pain is usually a lot more bearable at this stage compared to the first three days. It is harder during the first three days because you are low on energy at that stage. There will be periods where you will have a clear consciousness and feel great physically. Alternatively, you will also notice periods where you are weaker and heavier. Such periods are periods of deeper cleansing. Things change a lot during longer fasts. Things change from hour to hour, from day to day and the sequences do not follow any inherent logic. As such, in-depth analysis is of no use. You simply have to trust your body to know where to heal, how and what to detox and when to rest in between the more intensive segments of the fast.

Days 7-10: It's okay to undergo four- or five-day fasts. The benefits of fasting generally increase with every additional day of fasting. However, you should only extend your fast to the 7-10 part if you are emotionally ready to move beyond a three day fast. At this stage, you experience what is called a " healing crisis". This is a state where your body advances from basic detox and begins to uncover and heal deeper injuries, traumas, and illnesses.

A healing crisis will resemble a returning illness that is intensified during the fast. If you don't understand what's going on, you may be worried. The truth is everything you are going through at this point is perfectly normal. What occurs within your body at the point is this: the fasting procedure forces a deep-lying illness out of your body's physical depths and/or the subconscious of your mind. Its symptoms temporarily accompany the resurfacing of the said illness although they may be more acute than before. This may be an uncomfortable experience, but it is necessary to bring forth these illnesses to ensure your body heals and permanently expels them. This level of healing is unachievable using western medicine because toxic (allopathic) drugs and physical procedures simply suppress symptoms. This is not the same as dealing with the root causes of a given illness.

Extended Healing Fasts(14-40 days)

It seems surprising that fasting for two weeks or more is even a thing, right?

The proportion of people in the western world that will ever undertake an extended fast of 14 days or more is even smaller than the minuscule proportion of people in the western world that carry out a water fast. The reason for this? There is no need as occasional 7-10-day fasts accompanied by regular short fasts are enough to keep you healthy.

The deepest forms of healing can only be assessed through such long fasts as the extended fast. This healing can cure even the most serious illnesses deemed incurable by Western medicine. Contrary to what allopathic doctors tell you, conditions like chronic high blood pressure, multiple sclerosis, Type II diabetes, certain types of tumors as well as autoimmune disorders are all curable. They can be permanently healed through water fasting.

Only through extending the length of our fast can we experience the deepest spiritual cleansing. A reference point nowadays is the biblical 40-day fasts of Moses and Jesus even though other religions have demanded 40-day water fasts. It is said that even Pythagoras required potential students to carry out a 40 day fast as a prerequisite for his acceptance. We tend to dislike the idea of giving up food for an extended period; in actuality, it is just a matter of our unwillingness to forgo the pleasures and addictions of life. You shouldn't give in to the voices in your head that tell you that you will starve to death. As long as you are not severely malnourished and underweight, you have around 100,000 calories on you. The calories are trapped deep within your fat tissue, and they can only be released by ketosis. These calories are more than enough to last you for 40 days. You are able to even fast for much longer than 40 days if you are overweight even though this is not advisable.

On a basic level, the idea of an extended fast continues the process of the 7-10 day fast. The key difference is the extended fast is more powerful when it comes to the healing process associated with it which in this case, is the "healing crisis". A healing crisis initially occurs around the end of the first week of water fasting. It is characterized by the resurgence of symptoms of old traumas, illnesses and injuries before the afflictions in question are permanently expelled from the body. An identical process occurs at the end of the second week of water fasting, and this process is the main driving force behind the decision to extend a 7-10 day fast to make it at least 14 days. This process is the second healing crisis, and it causes even deeper issues that the first healing crisis couldn't reach. It heals and permanently expels any issues left from the first healing crisis. The meaning of all this is your body begins to tackle the more serious health issues from the beginning of the second week of water fasting. Before this point, your body has been removing the toxins that accumulated from everyday living especially for an individual that doesn't fast regularly.

At times, the most serious as well as the deepest health issues need healing crises that occur much later in the fast. "Much later " in this case can be 20, 30 or 40 days as there is no accurate way of predicting the time of its occurrence. You just have to trust your body as well as nature.

At times, healing will occur without a serious healing crisis. In cases like these, the symptoms of trauma or illness will abruptly vanish. When this happens, it's a sign that you have gotten rid of a health issue. Continuing the fast and knowing the best time to end the fast at this point is difficult. Situations like these give rise to the need for medical supervision while conducting an extended fast. Working with a professional also ensures you don't go beyond your body's nutritional capabilities while fasting.

Unless you feel there is a serious health issue buried within your body or you have a desire to reach your spiritual depths, there is no need for a fast exceeding the 7-10 day fast since a significant amount of healing and detox occurs during such a fast. For a healthy lifestyle, all you need are weekly 24- or 36-hour fasts (or regular intermittent fasting instead) combined with a 7-10 day fast from time to time. The frequency with which you undertake a 7-10 day fast is at your discretion. However, you shouldn't force your body to undergo such stress before it is ready even if you strongly feel it is the right thing to do. You can begin to trust your body once it has grown accustomed to the rigors of a 1-3 day fast because your body will know exactly what is best for you at this point. In fact, you will know when the time is right because you will feel an inner urge to do a 7-10 day fast and you will look forward to it. This urge comes once in a few years for some individuals while for some, it can come more than once in a given year. You just need to "listen" to your body.

There is a risk of a fast turning to starvation if you extend it indefinitely and this is a line you should never cross! At the point of starvation when even your fat stores are depleted, your body begins to break down your muscle tissue and internal organs. This can cause serious damage to you. The good thing is, your body will send you a very clear sign before any serious damage is done: extreme hunger. Two other scenarios should prompt you to end a fast. The first is a scenario whereby you deplete your muscle tissue before you deplete your fat reserves. Although ketosis is a very efficient process, it does not provide glucose which is essential as a fuel for the brain. Therefore, the glucose which can't be gotten from fat metabolism must be gotten from the depletion of muscles. The second scenario/ possibility is one where you run out of electrolytes (blood salts. This is a very dangerous situation to be in even though it is very unlikely. To prevent this scenario, you should get your blood tested at regular intervals after the initial 7 -10 days of fasting.

Variations of Water Fasting

The following are some of the most common ways to do an extended fast.

- **Strict Water Fasting.** Here, you only drink water, usually for several days in a row (typically no less than 24 hours).

- **Water plus non-caloric beverages.** This is a slight variation of water fast. In addition to drinking water, you can drink other non- caloric beverages like herbal tea and coffee (without milk, sugar or other sweeteners, including artificial non-caloric sweeteners).

- **Bone broth variation.** In this variation, you are allowed to consume a bone broth. A bone broth contains healthy fats and a lot of proteins, so this fast is not considered a true fast.

To experience good results, you can take bone broth, water as well as coffee and tea. If doing this provides results that you feel are desirable, you should continue the variant of the extended fast. "If you begin to get poor results with a bone broth or fat fasting, you can go to classic water-only fast."

- **Fat Fasting.** In this variant, you add healthy fats such as bulletproof coffee (black coffee with butter, coconut oil or MCT oil) in addition to water and non-caloric beverages. You also simply add the fat to your tea.

Chapter 5: Transitioning from a Regular Diet to Fasting

You can do a water fast if you are one of those people who eat until they are full one day and then easily avoid eating the following day. You don't need to plan it. However, you need to make plans for a smart transition into your next water fast if you are an individual who ends up eating an excessive amount of unhealthy food after a couple of days (or even hours) into your water fast.

Taking your time to plan and prepare for a water fast will greatly improve your chances of seeing the fast through till the end.

You need to get used to the idea of fasting before you start the real thing. Doing this enables you to transition to your next water fast properly.

You will discover that the fasting experience is a whole lot easier when you carry out a proper transition into full-blown water fast, you are also more likely to complete the required duration of the fast.

Reducing the size of your meals before you begin the fast is a major step in preparing yourself for a water fast.

You should eat most vegetables and fruits before beginning your fast. You should also eradicate processed foods, sugar and caffeine from your diet at least 2-3 days before your intended fast.

Before you begin your water fast, you should gradually reduce your portion sizes weeks before the commencement of your water fast. It is best if you do this at least a couple of days before you begin.

Intermittent fasting is also useful in making the transition to full water fast.

This can be simple as initially skipping food until noon every day. You will begin to skip food to 5 PM as you get closer to your fast. The time of your first meal will be at 7 PM and so on.

For someone who hasn't done a water fast before, this will provide you with a very good insight into the way things will be when you begin your water fast.

You might want to make a few adjustments before you begin water fast, especially if you find it difficult to stay away from food till 7 PM.

By the time of you get comfortable with the idea of skipping meals till 7 PM, your stomach, as well as your mind, are fully prepared to go completely without food.

It is possible to have a plan that is spread out over a month:

- Week 1: Skip breakfast

- Week 2: Skip both breakfast and lunch

- Week 3: Skip breakfast and lunch. You will also begin to decrease your dinner portions

- Week 4: Begin your water fast

What to Eat During the Transition Over to Water-Fasting

After the establishment of your healing metabolism, your digestive system will just have finished shutting down its day to day functions. Due to the temporary change, the majority of hunger pangs will begin to reduce in intensity after this point. Since your digestion has, in essence, come to a halt, it becomes very important for you to contemplate what and how you eat during the transition period before and after any fast that goes beyond three days.

To prevent your digestive system from shutting down with food being present in the intestines, you must ensure a proper transition to a fast. If the transition is not done properly, the remaining food will rot, and that is as uncomfortable as it sounds. The toxic by-products liberated from rotting food are detrimental to the body.

You will need to begin to change your eating habits around two or three weeks before the water fasting, and this is aimed at enhancing your nutrient uptake and familiarizing yourself with a healthy water fast.

- **Say goodbye to:** fast food, white flours, processed junk foods, processed meats, diet soda and drinks including regular soda, artificially and sugar-sweetened beverages and alcohol. You should also begin to keep off caffeine.

- **Say hello to:** Fresh juice with a variety of fruits and vegetables, salads, smoothies, soups as well as seeds, whole grains, natural nut butter, nuts, legumes, and beans. You should get used to drinking more water and enjoying the benefits of staying hydrated. Try to increase your water intake to 64 oz (2l) of water per day and add fresh orange, lemon or lime for flavor and vitamin C

- **Transition off animal proteins:** you should choose wild fish when possible as well as organic/pasture-raised eggs and reduce poultry consumption gradually during the week. If you are going to eat red meat, ensure it is lean, grass-fed, and don't eat beyond day 3 of the transition week.

- **Transition off dairy:** Ensure you choose organic dairy without added sugars. For non-dairy milk like almond, make sure it is unsweetened.

Gradually make the transition from cow's cheese to goat cheese once you get to the middle of the week. By the end of day 5, dairy should no longer be a part of your diet.

What to Drink During Fasting Without Breaking the Fast?

When engaging in water fasting, try to avoid all forms of caloric intake for some time. You're not supposed to eat food, desserts or snacks or even drink juices.

DUH! - It's a period where we starve!

At the point your body goes into a fasted state, your physiology changes into mild ketosis, which adds to fat burning and minimizes appetite. That is, the more you fast, the deeper you get into ketosis, it becomes easier.

However, we still have some additional beverages you can consume while fasting and won't end the fast. Factually, these beverages work to enhance the effectiveness of your fast as they empower cellular detoxification, cleansing of your gut and ketosis. What do you think is best to eat or drink while fasting?

Baking Soda. Although most people only use baking soda for cooking, it also has numerous health benefits unknown to many.

- It works for digestive problems
- It relieves bloating and constipation
- It helps to eliminate bad bacteria and parasites
- Lessens muscle soreness and fatigue
- Makes the acidity in the gut ineffective
- Enables the balance of pH levels available in the body

A teaspoon of baking could be added to your water for consumption to enhance physical performance and total well-being.

During the period of water-fasting, it is advisable to watch over your electrolytes because you tend to relieve yourself of minerals and water.

Baking soda contains 100% sodium bicarbonate, which is necessary to achieve some amount of sodium during fasting but, to be frank, it has an awful taste, so it is best used to curb hunger. Thankfully, after drinking it, you won't be left with an aftertaste, and you should be able to continue with your fast easier.

Glauber's Salts. When you aim to engage in water fasting for health reasons and to encourage cellular cleansing, then look into consuming Glauber's salt.

Glauber's salt serves as a mild laxative that activates bowel movements. By adding 5-20 grams of Glauber's salt into water, constipation can be eliminated, bloating can be minimized, and the digestive tract is left clean. Adding more to this amount could lead to diarrhea and can also cause dehydration, so remember not to overuse it.

Herbal Teas. Herbal teas have a wonderful taste and try to use it to stave off hunger during water fasting. As a bonus, they possess some detoxifying and various medicinal benefits as well.

- Chamomile helps to calm a worrying stomach and provide sleep

- Peppermint aids digestion lessens inflammation and muscle pain

- Jasmine empowers the immune system, curbs diabetes and lowers cholesterol

- Green tea is known as the healthiest drink after water in the world. It contains a great number of polyphenols that empowers heart and brain health. The small quantity of caffeine it contains helps to enhance fat burning.

- Black tea has enough compounds that help the heart, stress levels, and digestion.

Even though there are about 1-5 calories in a teacup, and it won't break you from the fasted state due to the small volume it contains.

Additionally, avoid brewing teas with fruit, berries or any other kinds of seasoning containing carbohydrates content. This is because the sugar in it will likely hold the beneficial advantages of autophagy.

Coffee. The simplest and best idea to suppress hunger during fasting is by drinking coffee because caffeine provides you with a jolt of energy and adds to your focus while enhancing fat burning.

Simultaneously, coffee possesses numerous health benefits like high polyphenol count, better blood sugar and lowered risk of Alzheimer's infection. So, it's a great booster for the mitochondria and brain.

To remain at a fasting state, continue to consume black coffee. Ordinarily adding a pinch of Stevia or Cinnamon, you could unknowingly end your fast. However, using a small quantity, like a few milligrams won't have any negative effect on your fasting. Also, instant coffee mixers possess some added ingredients that will end your fasted state.

Always be cautious of the amount of caffeine you drink.

Avoid consuming anything higher than 1-2 cups of coffee daily as it leads to caffeine intolerance and higher cortisol levels. Stress can stop you from ketosis but could as well prepare you to be more catabolic during fasting. Decaf, still, is potentially limitless, even though it contains caffeine also.

This makes me ask this question: Is it healthy to add butter to your coffee during fasting Bulletproof pattern?

Truly pure fat such as coconut oil, or MCT oil, butter, do not increase blood sugar; thus, it can put you in the semi-fasted mood. The fat won't go beyond the blood-brain barrier, and this will make your mind reason that it hasn't consumed anything.

However, this will hinder the process of autophagy even as the little amount of 50 calories keeps you into the fed mood and blocks the cell from self-digesting themselves.

Even though you'll lose some of the health benefits of detoxification, it's not an unhealthy thing, because it will equip you with energy and help you remain in ketosis.

From here, try to think of the reasons you're engaging in water fasting.

- If your reason for embarking on fasting is for weight loss and putting MCT oil or butter to your coffee is helpful to you then continue with it. Nevertheless, don't forget you'll need a small quantity intake of calories and adding all the sticks of butter into your cup will provide you with no less than one thousand calories.

- If your purpose is to clean your body against toxic proteins and inflammation carefully, then don't eat anything at all and engage in strict water fasting together with salt, mineral water, and teas.

Artificial Sweeteners. Is it possible to consume artificial sweeteners during water-fasting? Here lies the answer: It centers on the type of sweetener you're using, your reason for engaging in water fasting and how your system responds to them. So many sweeteners contain carbs in them, such as maltodextrin, dextrose or sucralose, try to avoid them.

Typical sweeteners such as Stevia doesn't have insulin or blood sugar, which makes them perfect for consumption.

Moreover, be cautious of how you specifically react to Stevia. Though it doesn't contain calories, it's 300 times sweeter than table sugar which could lead to placebo-like insulin response. That sweetness arouses your taste buds, which can make you end your fast - that's how powerful the mind is.

To make sure you don't fall into that trap, flee from all sweeteners during fasting, but if you can't, then test and experiment on them to see if it's suitable for your body.

Apple Cider Vinegar. Apple cider vinegar is a wonderful drink useful for fasting due to its anti-inflammatory and anti-bacterial compounds. It contains acidic substances but helpful in balancing your body's pH levels.

Apple cider vinegar has zero calories, and it possesses other minerals like potassium, iron and some amount of magnesium, suitable for fasting as it equips you to guide your electrolytes and curb deficiencies. Apple cider vinegar eliminates bad bacteria available in your gut and neutralizes hunger. Also, it can be joined with sparkling water to brew a fantastic tasty beverage.

Make sure to not take more than 1-2 tablespoons of ACV at a time to ensure you're not ending autophagy early.

Consuming it during your fasting period is okay and even better when breaking your fast. When breaking your fast put squeezed lemon juice to enhance the creation of digestive enzymes and ready your gut for eating. Try not to put lemon juice while fasting as it could pose the same placebo effect.

Mineral Water. Try to drink regular water, mineral, and sparkling water, because when you're engaging in fasting, you also flush out much water which may cause electrolyte imbalances and mineral deficiencies to your body. To avoid that, add a pinch of sea salt or pink Himalayan sea salt into your water. Additionally, when you consume ionized rock salt, it gives you iodine which encourages thyroid functioning and restricts hypothyroidism.

Help for Those New to Water Fasting

For decades, man has used this form of fasting for several reasons; however, this could be difficult at first for beginners, and that is the purpose of this section.

How to prepare for a fast

It is imperative to get your body prepped up for a fast before it commences. Intermittent fasting, as well as KD for a period of 2-3 weeks, is a good way to start. As your body gradually adapts to the new way of living, you can then extend the fasting period.

Just like a muscle, the more you train it, the bigger and stronger it becomes. So also, the more you fast, the easier it becomes. This is known as fasting fitness.

Another way to prep the body for what lies ahead is to go on a 20-24 hour fast weekly for a minimum of 1-2 weeks before commencing on the water fasting period. This strategy will help your body adapt to periods of abstinence from food.[27]

Cut down your schedule to have a low-stress level. Stress, especially at a high level, is one of the most discouraging factors while fasting. Therefore, it is expedient that you arrange your schedule in such a way that it becomes so light and you will still have time to rest and even take a vacation. This is very necessary especially at the early stages of water fasting when the body is just getting used to a new way of living. However, after developing a sufficient amount of fasting stamina, keep yourself engage to stay distracted especially when hunger sets in. Also, when the body is utilizing a large number of ketones, you are more active and productive.

If after trying so hard to adjust your schedule you still found out that you just can't escape from a high level of stress, then extended water fast is not ideal for you. You can try taking short and deep breaths once or twice daily.

Taking in short and deep breaths daily has a lot of health benefits. Short breaths boost the production of adrenaline as well as other fight and flight hormoncs which slows down the process of healing. Long and deep breath, however, produces the opposite effect by stimulating the healing process.

Try as much as possible to avoid negative people. There are two sets of people we are likely to come across in life:

- Positive people who encourage us to be the best that we can.

- Negative people who try as much as possible to drag you down.

You need to stay away from the second group of people during a fast as they could weaken your determination.

If such negative people are unavoidable (family member or workmates) why not sit them down and have a heart-heart discussion with them. However, try not to act as a judge in the matter. Rather, explain your goals and the importance of the exercise to them. You could be surprised at the effect of such conversation as they may suddenly become supportive.

Drink a lot of filtered water. Particularly if you are on an extended fast, hydration is vital. The reason is that your body depletes its sugar reservoir in the form of glycogen stored in the liver and muscles, so you lose water as well. Glycogen is lost alongside water, and once you deplete this source of energy, you will pass out the excess water. Also, the reduction in the levels of your insulin results in the excretion of additional sodium, and this would help your body to lose more water.

You would require access to enough clean water. It would be very helpful to get a very quality reverse osmosis system such as the Big Berkely water system or the iSpring that would make clean water easily available in your home. If this would not be possible, you can also buy bottled Fiji water from a nearby grocery store.

It is important to have a personal water system and drinking glasses or mason jars to lower the risk of plastic exposure. The Big Berkey and iSpring are inexpensive, and after a few months, the cost is lower, compared to buying the bottled Fiji water. Your goal should be to drink at least one ounce of water for every pound of your weight.

Get Some Quality Salts. While on an extended fast, electrolytes are required, and I recommend using high-quality salts like Himalayan Sea Salt, Celtic Sea Salt, and Redmond's Real Salt.

Like I earlier said, your insulin levels are reduced when you are fasting. Insulin is a hormone that functions in driving sugars into the body cells, and it also causes sodium retention. Reduced levels of insulin cause sodium to be excreted in high quantities.

When you start feeling light-headed or tired during the fast, place a pinch of salt on your tongue, then drink about 4 to 8 ounces of water. There is an instant increase in brain function and energy for most people.

Fix a spa day. Fasting helps you to save money since you won't be eating, I would advise that you rechannel that money to yourself. Schedule an appointment or two at the spa, enjoy the sauna, or get a message. All these can decrease stress, rid your body of toxins and make your fast less stressful.

As humans, we are naturally predisposed to gravitate towards pleasurable activities. One way we can do this is through food, and this is the reason a lot of us battle with food addictions. It is also the reason we usually feel a wide range of emotions while on a water fast. Our bodies have adapted to the neurochemical spike we get from food, so it would be difficult to adjust to the absence of this each day.

Fixing one or two spa days gives your body something positive to expect as a reward. You would be amazed at how this simple act can help you satisfy those emotions that you might experience in the course of the fast. The spa treatment causes you to expect something very nice as a form of personal reward.

If you can, avoid the kitchen. One of the major things most people have to battle against if they enter the kitchen is food cravings. I usually suggest that they try as much as possible to stay away from the kitchen. This is particularly important when you start fasting for the first time. After some time, you become mentally strong enough to avoid this temptation.

If it is impossible to stay away from the kitchen, get drinking water, or prepare herbal tea and make sure that you are drinking this while cooking in the kitchen. Drinking the water helps to suppress hunger and cravings for food.

Strategize your drinking times. Usually, you experience increased hunger at your usual feeding times. This is a natural and expected process that is caused by ghrelin, which is the hormone that is responsible for making you hungry. When you drink water, the level of ghrelin is lowered, resulting in lower levels of hunger as well. You can also consider drinking herbal teas like chamomile or green tea.

Take a fruity drink. If you are feeling very low during your course of water fasting, consider making a zero-calories lemonade by mixing liquid stevia and organic lemon juice to water. Drinking this mix would produce a boost in the neurotransmitters that would lift your mood; thus, making your water fast more fun.

Drinking a fruity drink is one of the things I enjoy doing most because it positively lifts my mood and makes the fast less uncomfortable and more enjoyable. My family and I enjoy the new natural water Stevia that is rich in fruit, and it is also excellent when added to water. You only need a little bit since it is very sweet and has zero calories or sugar.

Allow your feet to touch the ground every day. It can be particularly beneficial to make you put your bare feet on sand, grass or dirt. The Earth has some anions (negative ions) and rich electromagnetic frequency that can serve as antioxidants. We are unable to absorb anions due to the rubber soles on our shoes.

Walking in socks or barefoot on the Earth helps you to activate your body's electromagnetic current and feel enhanced energy, mental alertness, and relaxation. This is similar to having a bath and washing away all the Electromagnetic field that your body might have absorbed. Like a lot of us that like taking a bath or shower every day, it would be nice to cleanse your electromagnetic field every day by contact with the bare floor for 10 minutes or more.

It would be simpler to do this in warmer climates, compared to colder climates. Consider wearing socks or walking around your neighborhood when it is cold outside. Your neighbors might think you are a little odd, but the outcome would be pleasing. If you can afford to, you could also take a vacation to a hot, sunny beach for your fast when it is winter, and there are lots of snow.

If daily grounding isn't possible, don't worry, your fast would still be effective. Daily grounding would only make your fast less discomforting.

If you can, get sunshine every day. It is very helpful to get your body in the sun, although, make sure that you avoid getting a sunburn while catching that extra sunshine. A suntan enhances vitamin D and improves fat depletion that tilts your body system into ketosis.

Additionally, the sun has strong biophotons that can lower stress hormones and cause the production of excitatory neurotransmitters like dopamine, serotonin, and endorphins that would make you enjoy your fasting process more.

If you can afford to, this is an additional reason to take a vacation to the beach for your initial fast. Obviously, not all individuals can afford to do this, but you can still achieve excellent outcomes while fasting even in the absence of the sun, it only makes it even more enjoyable.

Set your body in motion. It can be extremely beneficial to go out and take walks all through the day. By nature, walking enhances the lymphatic and circulatory systems and increases excitatory neurotransmitters.

It is more advisable to take walks in a place filled with plants like the woods or a park so that you can get a contra-natural electromagnetic field from nature. If it is impossible or you are restricted by the weather, then take a walk in your home. You can also walk to and from the store, use a bike, treadmill or elliptical.

Your aim is not to use up your calories or work out. Walking is only a leisurely exercise to set your body in motion at a comfortable speed. The goal is to get a minimum of 40 to 60 minutes of leisurely movement every day divided into sections all through the day. You can divide it into 10 minutes- 4 to 6 times every day, 15 minutes- 3 to 4 times every day, or 20 minutes- 2 to 3 times every day. Select the method that would be suitable and convenient for you.

Fix relaxation periods. In the world today, we are constantly moving, and this makes us 'efficiency' addicts. Water fast enables you to live contrary to the way that we have become addicted to and allows you periods of rest, take a quick nap, have a warm bath, use some essential oils and to just enjoy yourself.

If you are water fasting for the first time, you might require additional rest compared to when you have been fasting intermittently for some time or if you have done at least one extended fast. With time, while you develop your fasting habit, and you notice that you are very efficient while water fasting, it might even be a better idea to engage yourself in pleasurable activities so that you would not have to think about food.

You are permitted to be busy when fasting only when you have adjusted, and you are beginning to enjoy it, but when you start feeling weak and tired, it is advisable to slow down and rest.

Chapter 6: Understanding your Fasting Routine

Finding the Most Suitable Eating Routine

If you are usually very busy, and you are always on the go, the most effective habit to adopt is one that you can adhere to and that you know you can accomplish. Even if there might be a daily variation in your fasting routine, it has to be effective enough for your lifestyle.

Consider how your days go and what would be most effective. For instance:

- 16-hour fasts on Monday, Wednesday and Friday

- 18-20 hour fasts on Tuesday, Thursday and Saturday, since you would be busier

Try not to worry excessively about your fasting and eating times. You might not feel like eating even when it is time to eat some times, if this happens, continue your fast.

One of the challenges of fasting that is hardly talked about is understanding how to handle yourself to the best of your capabilities. This is where the phrase, "different strokes for different folks" comes to play, so it is not realistic to recommend a particular method for everyone to use to enhance their energy and effectiveness. One thing that can be done by everyone to improve the efficacy and energy when on a fast is to manipulate your morning routine until you discover an effective method. This would be beneficial in getting the best out of your morning routine for optimum effectiveness and energy. There is no one-size-fits-all strategy. Discover the hours that are effective for your lifestyle and start with that.

As soon as you wake up, meditate for 15 minutes

Each morning, as soon as you get out of bed, place a pillow on the ground and sit on it, then engage in 15 minutes of meditation. It is quite hard to clear your mind while sitting since thinking of suppressing a thought is another form of thinking too. It might take time to be skilled at it, but as soon as you are, it can be very beneficial in ways like enhancing your capability to think, managing stress better, being more attentive and making rational decisions. Science has also proved that your brain can be improved physically through meditation. It does this by reducing the grey-matter in the amygdala, and this helps to reduce stress and worry, at the same time, the grey matter in the hippocampus-which is the area of memory and learning is increased.

Morning workouts: how to do it

If you prefer to work out in the morning, how do you handle working out while fasting? The problem with exercising in the morning is that you might lose muscle mass. The reason for this is that your body starts using up your muscle once protein is no longer available. Buying BCAAs is a waste of money because they do not help you gain or maintain your muscle and make sure to follow comfortable and light exercise routines. If you prefer workout after your workday, like in the evening, then working out while fasting shouldn't be a problem. It is an individual choice to eat before working out. Ensure that you still have carbs to energize you before exercising. If your dinner is two hours or more before exercising, eat protein together with carbs such as oats or sweet potato that takes a while to digest. If it would be less than two hours, you must eat a meal that digests easily. Fruits like banana or apple together with one protein scoop is an excellent idea. You should make your fasting routine to fit your lifestyle.

Establish a routine

Water Fasting entails going without food and taking only water for a certain period- from 12 hours to 40 days or more. To sustain their health, most people who fast regularly, fast for 24 hours once a week. Intermittent fasting is also practiced widely. There is a misconception that intermittent fasting causes weakness. This is untrue.

In contrast, it enhances your energy and health. After intermittent fasting, your energy level increases. At the beginning of your fast, your body stimulates the pituitary gland to secrete HGH (Human Growth Hormone). The increase in hormone makes your body to utilize additional fat as a fuel source, rather than degrading your muscle. There is no proof that a 72-hour fast would lower your muscle mass. If your weight reduces, it is as a result of fat reduction. A 24-hour fast is enough to sustain your health and energy. However, what happens in the case of a chronic health issue that requires a solution? Here, you would have to engage in long-term fasts that might range from 3 to 21 days, or even more. With the supervision of a professional, most illnesses can be cured by fasting moderately.

Planning the lengths of your fasts

Fix a timeframe for your water fast. Try starting with a 24-hour fast. If you are fasting alone, restrict your water fast to 3 days. There is some proof that fasting for a short period like 1-3 days is beneficial to health. If you would be fasting for a more extended period, ensure that it is under the guidance of a medical expert, like at a fasting retreat where a chiropractor or a medical expert can guide you. It might be less risky. Instead of long-term fasts for more than three days, periodic short-term fasts might be more beneficial. Try doing a water fast once a week.

Guidelines for fasting length and period

You can use Time Blocking to establish your routines. Time Blocking is when you fix a block of time for every meal period. I refer to this as 'directing your time.' Majority of the time, the instant we become adapted to fasting and no longer experience hunger pangs while fasting, eating becomes what we do only out of boredom. Or when we have a craving, or maybe time is moving too slow.

We tend to monitor the clock, asking ourselves: "How many hours left? Really, I can't eat for another 4 hours? How is that possible?" Time Blocking becomes essential here. This was the approach I frequently used in the early weeks of my fast, during the transitional phase of a ketogenic diet or intermittent fasting

These are a few tips for using Time Blocking when on a water fast

Plan your day one- or two-hour sections, make your primary task or activity for each time frame in a bullet format. You can do this with colorful highlighters or pens.

It is not necessary to be precise about what you have to do for each hour. It is acceptable to make non-specific statements about the things that you want to achieve.

Doctors recommend drinking extra water whether you are fasting or not so be mindful to include this. Include any multivitamins that might have been recommended by your doctor. Multivitamins and water would go a long way.

Make sure to include your fasting hour.

Ensure that your Block List is close to you at every time of the day and highlight or cancel out each block that represents a complete task. Since you now have a sense of direction, time would pass much faster, and you will be amazed by your effectiveness and cognizance

This is very effective for people who are homeschooled, corporate workers and homemakers, even those who have free work days. It is particularly beneficial to amateurs in water fasting and for a lengthier fasting period.

Longer is greater: advantages of Fasting for up to 3 days

When fasting, longer is better, although your goals will determine how long you fast. It is not better generally, but for longevity, protection against cancer, stronger immunity, and anti-aging, it can be a good option. Walter Longo, a prolific USC researcher, has carried out extensive research on the 'stronger immunity' benefit.

In Longo and his colleague's research published in Cell,[28] they explained the primary metabolic events after long periods of 3-day fasts. Participants produced additional white blood cells- that implies improved immunity, after 3 days. The benefit of protection against cancer was discovered too. Longo discovered that both cancer patients who were undergoing therapy and healthy people benefited health-wise, after fasting for 3 days. Like other cells in the body, cancer cells get nourishment from glucose, fasting deprives cancer cells of glucose, resulting in their deaths and this can help to protect against cancer later.

Limiting calorie intake every day helps to rid the body of the by-products of cells, fasting for 3-5 days uses up the entire glycogen in the body, thereby clearing even more by-product from the cells.

Strategies for Extended Fasting

There are unlimited methods to reap the benefits of fasting, and I will be discussing some of this that pertains to extended fasting:

- Modern- this strategy infuses caffeine in addition to some multivitamins

- Minimalist- this strategy involves salts- as a source of electrolytes and water

They are both beneficial, but this is determined by how determined you are to follow the rules of extended fasting.

Minimalist Strategy. As the name suggests, the minimalist fasting strategy is minimal. It simulates a primitive period perfectly. There was no caffeine for our forefathers to use to suppress hunger, and neither was there BCAA (Branched Chain Amino Acid) to prevent loss of muscle. Although a few advocates of fasting suggest that caffeine does not stop the fast, one cup of coffee will inhibit some fasting processes. Also, BCAAs generate a response to insulin, which would inhibit some other fasting processes. This strategy involves going without foods, exclusively drinking water (while including a pinch of salt), and no multivitamins at all

Modern Strategy. This strategy infuses some modern inventions while producing the benefits of long-term fasting. It involves tea and coffee, which have the least possible calories and also represses hunger. This makes fasting easier for people who might feel intense hunger pangs.

A few people use supplements like BCAAs and exogenous ketones. Exogenous ketones stimulate the process of utilizing ketones (gotten from fat) as a fuel source and BCAAs prevent muscle loss.

Make sure to select the exogenous ketone carefully that you would be using; the most popular ketone is BHB (Beta-hydroxybutyrate)

which contains MCT powder that is enriched with calories and can bring you out of your fast.

Suggested Timetable for Water Fasts

- Stage 0- One week of a reduced normal diet

- Stage 1- At least two weeks of low-fat cleansing diet

- Stage 3- Drink water exclusively for 3-5 days.

- Stage 4- 1-4 days of steamed vegetables, miso soup, and fresh fruit juice.

- Stage 5- 5-14 days of a low-fat cleansing diet

Timetable for 3-day Fast

A 3-day fast might appear more challenging than it really is. The hardest part of a 3-day fast is stopping the fast at the end (we will discuss this later)

This timetable was constructed based on Tim Ferriss' experience. Going on 70% of the fast during the weekend may prevent disruptions in your work days during the week.

- 8pm, Thursday- Round up your last meal and start your fast.

- 8am, Friday- For 3-4 hours, start walking. Doing this uses up your glycogen reserves and helps to change your energy source for glucose to fat. If you prefer to drink coffee first, do so, it might be helpful. While walking, you could listen to audiobooks or make a call

- Friday/Saturday - If you are free to go on extended walks at any time, go. Total depletion of glycogen reserves takes 28-48 hours, though this is determined by your experience and diet. The process is faster when you walk for more extended periods.

NOTE: Ensure that you are drinking enough water, but not excessively. Drink water only when you are thirsty. Drinking too much water might wash away a lot of electrolytes from your body. To prevent this too, include a pinch of salt. The most difficult part of going on a 3-day fast is not the hunger pangs but ending the fast.

Return to Normal: Regular Diet

Individual requirements, emotional, physical and spiritual state determines the period that would be spent on these stages to prepare and recover from water fasting.

NOTE: One day of water fasting is equal to one day of recovery, if you engage in water fasting for ten days, then you should rest for a minimum of 10 days before any intense activity.

End of the Day routine and meditation (coupled with meditation techniques)

Yoga, together with meditation at the end of the day will improve your mood. A few of the best yoga practices can happen when you have no food in your system. You might even sense your internal organs as you dig deeper and tap into the meditation during yoga while you are fasting. You don't have to feel like your energy is insufficient for yoga, it is good to do something mild, but if you regularly practice yoga, it feels nice to twist the spaces that do not exist on a normal day in your body. While on a fast, meditation can be more intense. It is exciting to sense your mind becoming peaceful very fast, like turning in a switch. If you are regularly eating, it might take a minimum of half the time spent during a one-hour meditation to experience the peace; whereas, if you are fasting, it is easier to experience the peace while meditating, and achieve the feeling of 'nothing' that experienced yogis reach with equal experience and silence

You can engage in the following activities:

- Spine Healing Session.

- Yoga Nidra Session

- Sound Healing Therapy

- Transformational Breathing Therapy

- Thai Box and Chi

- Mandala Painting Session

When your internal organs are left to rest, without expending energy on digestion, there is a more intense cleansing that leads to cell renewal. It is similar to pressing a reset button internally. There is improved absorption of vitamins and minerals that reduce the space that food can be absorbed while getting an equal feeling of satiety and health benefits. This period is also beneficial for tissues and glands producing smooth skin and clearer eyes.

Chapter 7: Ending the Water Fasting Process the Proper Way

Since you won't be consuming solid food while embarking on a water fast, your digestion might not be able to handle your regular diet at the beginning. When you eat too many hard-to-digest foods after breaking your water fast, it could lead to devastating outcomes.

Below is a list of foods you can follow to easily and properly break a water fast and shun any potential complications within the process.

- Fruit juice

- Vegetable juice

- Raw fruit and green leafy vegetables

- Yogurt

- Vegetable soup and cooked vegetables

- Cooked grains and beans

- Milk, dairy, and eggs

- Meat, fish, and poultry

Everything Else

The listed foods are orderly arranged on how challenging they will be to digest. At the top of the list are the easily digestible ones, while the difficult-to-digest ones are listed at the bottom.

After breaking your water fast, endeavor to start with the foods at the top of the list and gradually move down to the hard ones. You can add more foods from the list, with every meal.

For example: End the water fast using orange juice, which is found in group list #1, later on, eat a banana which is #3. When you find out that your system is okay, prepare a small amount of salad and top it with yogurt, as you can see in food groups #4 and #5 as the next food in line.

Endeavor to break your fast with a small number of meals making sure to leave two hours of space apart. After adding food continuously to the list, you can begin increasing the number of your meals.

If your fasting lasted for two days, it's possible you won't have any issues when you end your fast, and there shouldn't be any issues with going back to your old diet right from the beginning. However, if your fasting lasted for a week or more, then it will take time to transition back into your normal diet pattern gradually.

The overall rule is, the more hours you fasted, the wiser and more cautious you should be when ending the fast. Irrespective of how little the time you take to fast is, there won't be any problem if you take time to get back to your normal diet easily.

However, depending on the hours you fasted, it could take you from 1-4 days before your digestion can be 100% in order again.

The simple truth is, not everybody will follow the laid down guide provided, it's fine to skip one or two during the process, but it's healthier to keep it in mind as a general guide.

Things to Avoid Drinking and Eating When Ending Your Fast

Stay away from fried foods or anything with much oil, or even added fats as they're difficult to digest.

Avoid all high-carbohydrate foods; like pizza, pasta, white rice, and bread. Carbohydrate foods not only have zero calories, but they also affect blood sugar levels. A quick change in blood sugar levels will affect the smoothness of your fasting and will harm the benefits attached to fasting, like fat loss and added insulin sensitivity.

Avoid anything containing refined or processed sugars; content such as high fructose corn syrup, table sugar, and agave nectar. The way you're trying to shun filling your caloric limits during your fasting periods with empty calories, ensure you don't rubbish those 500 or 600 calories on simple sugars.

In fulfilling your sweet tooth, try honey and maple syrup which are two sweeteners that are good choices when consumed at moderation. Also, processed sugars are to be avoided in those two days a week you'll engage in fasting. If staying away from sugar is difficult, try remembering that it's only twice a week you'll be going without it.

Furthermore, avoiding sugar intake twice-a-week will help you combat sugar addiction.

Add sweetener and other additives to your coffee with caution. Although only one cup of black coffee contains five insignificant calories, 260 calories can be gained from drinking one 16oz. Mocha- if the whipped cream is included, that cup of coffee becomes 330 calories.

Avoid sports drinks, regular soda, juices, or diet soda. It is usual for most Americans to get about 140-180 calories every day from sweet beverages such as sports drink and soda. Stay away from the diet forms too.

Alcohol. In a 2012 research, it was discovered that Americans drink alcoholic beverages that contain about 300 calories each day. This might appear insignificant but think about the accumulated value gotten in one week. However, a lot of people even drink more than that every day.

One hundred twenty-five calories are contained in one 5-oz glass of red wine. One standard 12-oz beer has caloric content higher than 125, and diet cola and double vodka contains an alarming 258 calories. Indulging in any of these drinks can increase your caloric restrictions on the days when you are fasting.

Unhealthy foods such as pretzels, chips, buttery popcorn, candy, fruit snacks, etc. One of the numerous advantages of fasting is the purification of the body. Eating unhealthy foods which are notably filled with ingredients that are deficient in some nutrients while fasting will, in reality, produce more poisons in addition to the ones your body is trying to eliminate. Rather than eating these unhealthy foods, eat only natural, whole or unpackaged foods when you are fasting as well as ending a fast.

Eating After a Water Fast

A few people engage in this type of fasting to improve their health- weight loss or toxin elimination. Others use water fasting to get a clear head and enter into the state of meditation. Regardless of the purpose of the fast, the fast would come to an end, and you will have to start eating. It doesn't matter if your fast is only short-term, be careful of when you begin eating again.

Step 1: On the morning of the day after your fast ended, mix one part water with one part fruit or vegetable and drink. If you can, use a juicer to produce your juice. The less concentrated juice would provide nourishment without causing a disturbance in your digestive system.

Step 2: On the afternoon of the day after your fast ended, drink one cup of chicken broth or vegetable. If you like, eat plain crackers or a piece of bread together with the broth. Keep drinking the juice mix. The soup provides additional nourishment and primes your digestive system for normal foods.

Step 3: On the evening of the day after your fast ended, drink a more substantial soup like minestrone or vegetables. Eat a bit of undressed salad together with vegetables and fresh fruits. Consume one glass of juice that is not diluted with water.

Step 4: On the second day after your fast ended, keep eating the vegetables and fresh fruits, juices, and fruits. In the evening, you can include dairy products like yogurt or milk.

Step 5: On the fourth day, continue with your regular feeding routine. Beginning from the third or fourth day, start including other whole foods that are cooked like meat, fish, nuts, eggs, whole grains and uncooked fruits and vegetables. Ensure that your legumes and grains are cooked thoroughly since this is to soften them and make them easily digestible. On the fifth day, you are free to include non-cultured dairy products like milk, and meat or eggs. Ensure that your meals contain low-fat so that you do not overwhelm your digestive system. Though it is usually recommended, cooked vegetables, fresh juices, and organic fruits are unnecessary.

How Long the Gradual Process Should Take to Get Back to "Normal"

Due to the dormancy of your digestive system, the transit from a fast is very significant. Your system is still unable to digest, but you have to gradually revive it, reverently, by consuming foods that are easy to digest in tiny portions. If not, it would be very uncomfortable. The same way the remnant of food in the gut at the start of long-term fast decay, it can happen in this case too. Except for basic fruits and vegetables, or juices, any other food remains in the stomach, till your digestive system is capable of digesting. This process may take days to finish. After a fast, the period of restoration of healthy feeding with a regular appetite is as long as the duration of the actual fast.

When ending a water fast, constipation might result in the first few days. Constipation happens due to the sharp increase in fiber and food consumption. To lower the risks of constipation, drink adequate fluids around 6-8 oz. Glasses of fluid every day all through the day and slowly increase food consumption. Make sure to avoid going back to your previous fasting habits. Fasting would be less beneficial for your health if you go back to consuming meals rich in fat and sugar later. The health advantages of your fast can be maintained by eating a low-sodium diet that is high in whole grains, fruits or vegetables, or a diet low in fat.

Engage in 30 minutes of a workout five days a week. Adopt a healthy lifestyle to enhance your health and general wellness, allocate only a small portion to fasting.

Chapter 8: Tips and Tricks Water Fasting Success

Relationship Between Autophagy and Ketogenic Diet

Some things are dependent on one another such as water fasting, the ketogenic lifestyle, and autophagy. One of the more popular methods of activating autophagy is by undergoing a ketogenic diet.

Before proceeding, it is essential to note that the Ketogenic Diet does not enhance your capability to go without eating- every machine requires an energy source. The mechanism by which keto works is by providing your body with a method of using a more persistent energy source obtained from heavy fats instead of carbohydrates. Normally, people who are not used to the Ketogenic Diet experience hunger pangs when they do not eat snacks for a few hours. These hanger pangs can be regularly seen in people that are dependent on quickly depleted carbs. If you already have previously adapted to keto, you should be able to function without food for days and without any need to eat.

Fasting lowers the level of insulin and blood sugar which promotes the secretion of hormones that deplete fats, like adrenaline and glucagon. This then supports the degradation of fats known as triglyceride reserves in adipose tissue. Eventually, when triglycerides are transported to the liver, they are used as a source of fuel or to generate ketone bodies. Once your ketone levels become about 7-8 mmol/L that's when you know your body has begun ketosis.[29]

As a result of reduced carbohydrate intake, the ketogenic diet results in a decrease in the levels of insulin and glucose. Contrary to fasting, some amount of protein and foods rich in fats are permitted. Unlike glucose, fats and proteins do not significantly affect the levels of blood glucose.

Contrarily, fat does not have this effect, eating a diet rich in fat, but low in protein and carbs divert your energy source to ketone bodies and imitates a natural, fasted condition. This means that by being in a ketotic state, you would be stimulating autophagy.[30]

Furthermore, lowering your intake of protein and carbohydrates, in turn, lowers the number of poisonous substances that are absorbed by your body, so there is just a little toxin for your body to eliminate, making autophagy even more fully effective.

This is probably why people that engage in the keto diet start feeling like an improved version of themselves. Their bodies are eliminating toxins, and there is an upgrade in their health.

One of the main proponents of the ketogenic diet is water fasting because digesting even the healthiest meals uses energy and can stress the body eventually. Water fasting helps the body to rest and permits recycling of excess energy.

Additionally, the body enters into a ketotic state more rapidly if you are on a water fast. Water fasting creates extended, more efficient periods of ketosis. Also, a more intense restoration at cellular levels is observed while on a water fast.

Even though this is similar to what happens on a Ketogenic Diet, but water fasting makes the process faster with the additional advantages we have discussed previously.

The type of fat used to generate ketones is one other difference between water fasting and a keto diet. Fat reservoirs are the source of fat when you are on a fast. However, the fat in keto is gotten from the high-fat meals you are consuming. The quantity of calories gotten from your dietary fat determines if a ketogenic diet would result in weight loss.

Start Fasting Gradually

It might be challenging to undergo a water fast, but your body starts to adapt to the recent changes eventually. Within the first three days, you might be tempted to stop. The smell of food excites you, and you will start to imagine all the foods you would get to eat after breaking your fast. By day three, ketosis is complete, and you will start to feel dizzy if you get up too fast, have intense headaches, and sleep disturbances.

After two weeks, you would no longer feel the intense headaches and hunger pangs. You might still feel dizzy and very cold because the levels of your blood pressure are still lower than normal. By then you can easily cook family meals without temptations, and you would begin to detest the smell of sugary snacks and unhealthy foods.

In comparison to the first two weeks, the third week should be easier because this is because the body is adapting to the recent changes and you have eliminated the majority of the toxins in your body lowering flu-like and discomforting after effects.

Begin with a small fast. How many hours can you go without food? Three hours? Six hours? Begin with that and gradually add one hour every day.

Remember: Before you start running – learn to walk first.

Most people make the common error of starting directly with 24-hour fasts when they are used to 3-6 meals each day together with snacks. In some cases, it is possible to attempt this, but it might begin to feel like torture and starvation.

Eating the Right Foods

On fasting days, eat a little bit of food. Generally, fasting entails partially or completely going without food or drinks for a certain period.

Though it is possible to exclude food completely on fasting days, a few fasting strategies such as the 5:2 diet permits you to eat about 25% of your calorie needs in one day.[31]

If you are thinking of starting a fast, limit your caloric intake to enable yourself to eat small quantities during your fasting days. Limiting your intake can be healthier than engaging in a complete fast when you're starting as a beginner.

This method might help to lower the risks of fasting like experiencing hunger, inability to concentrate or light-headedness.

Because you do not feel really hungry, it might also make it easier to continue with the fast.[32]

Ensure Adequate Hydration. It is important to drink sufficient amounts of liquid while on a fast because thirst, fatigue, headaches, and dry mouths can be caused by mild dehydration.

Many health experts advise people to use the 8 by 8 rule- 8 glasses that are 8 oz. in size (less than 2 liters) of liquid each day- to ensure adequate hydration.

Although this might be enough, the quantity of liquid you need depends on you as an individual. It is very easy to become dehydrated while fasting because 20-30% of the fluid required by your body comes from food.

While fasting, a lot of people try to drink 2-3 liters (8.5-13 cups) of water throughout the day. But, thirst should guide you on when it is time to drink additional water, follow the instructions that your body is telling. Only you know when too much water is too much.

Eat Plenty of Protein. For most people, fasting is a form of weight loss although you have to remember that a reduction in caloric intake will make you lose not just fat but muscle as well.

One method of reducing the risk of losing muscle while on a fast is to make sure that you are consuming sufficient amount of proteins on the days that you are allowed to eat food.[33]

Also, adding protein to the small-sized meals on your fast days can help suppress your hunger and provide other beneficial effects.

Some researchers propose that getting 30% of your calories by eating protein can significantly suppress your appetite.[34]

Because of this, some bad after effects of fasting can be reduced by consuming some form of good protein.

Avoid ending your Fasts With large Meals. After fasting for a while, the thought of ending your fast with a large meal can be enticing but ending you fast with a large meal can make you weak and bloated. Also, if you desire to lose weight, large meals might impede your fasting objectives by impeding or stopping your weight loss process.

Eating too many calories after a fast lowers your caloric deficit because your total caloric intake affects your health, so the most effective way of ending a fast is to keep eating normally and continue with your usual eating schedule

Exercise while fasting. Before starting any workout routine, consult your doctor, especially when you are fasting. Your doctor knows your medical history and can specifically advise you on what to do. Also, tell your doctor about your wish to fast and your workout routine, so your doctor would know if this is suitable or unsafe.

Stop the fast and workout if you experience any discomfort or pain when exercising, or the aftereffects of a fast, and you are advised to call your doctor instantly. Your doctor would decide if your heart can cope with exercises when you are on a fast.

How does it feel to workout while fasting? This is determined by many factors, ranging from the fasting approach you use to the response of your body has to the fast. Following your body's directions is pertinent. If fasting makes you too tired to exercise, solve your nutrition issues first, then you can exercise later.

Although safety should be your priority, a number of exercise routines can enhance fasting.

Schedule your meals around your exercises. Cardio can be done on an empty stomach. You are allowed to go on a jog or register for that early morning spin session. However, it is vital to select the right foods before you attempt any form of cardio.

Since you know you would be working out, you should carefully select what to eat on the previous day as determined by how hard you would be exercising. For instance, you may want to increase your glycogen reserves by eating complex carbohydrates for dinner, the previous night so that you would be provided with easily accessible energy for your cardio exercise. It is inadvisable to do cardio when your stomach is full because the muscle's abrupt demand for blood diverts the important blood required for nutrient digestion and absorption. The best thing is to make plans beforehand to ensure that your nutrition provides the nutrients for your intense exercise, even though you would be exercising the following morning.

Exercise Suggestions For You

Choose less stressful exercises. While on a fast, a simple exercise might be very helpful because it makes sure that your body does not convert protein to an energy source.

While fasting, your body is dependent on energy reserved in the form of glycogen (this is the form in which glucose is stored by your body) If it has been a while since you last ate, your glycogen reserved might have been depleted, this would drive your body to use protein as a source of energy.

- Rather than working out by running, walk. Moderate walks are a less stressful way of increasing your heart rate.

- Engage in Tai Chi or light yoga. Gradual, precise movements stabilize and enhance your body, and this old approach is a popular way of clearing and soothing the mind.

- Engage in light yard chores or gardening. Gardening needs you to lift, bend or move in other ways. Yard work and gardening are both excellent activities that mimic exercise.

However the intense exercise may be, the moment you start to feel dizzy or weak, stop the exercise instantly. You might have to drink water and eat a small portion of food to bring your energy level back up.

The great thing is that engaging in less stressful workouts while fasting makes the body to start using fat as a source of energy. For people that are trying to lose weight, this is very beneficial.

Make sure your workout routine is practical. Rather than walking, you might feel like running, or you might feel that you can cope with lifting heavy weights. However, fasting alters the normal limits of your body.

If your fast is for a religious purpose, or a medical reason, make plans to include less stressful workouts that you can easily do. You can continue with your regular workout routine as soon as your fast has ended.

If your fast extends from dusk to dawn, you have to stay away from working out during those periods and make sure to workout at a time that is close to your eating periods in the morning or evening.

If the purpose of your fast is to lose weight or other health reasons, you have to include exercises with caution. Take care to do less stressful workouts on your fasting days, and engage in rigorous exercises on days that you eat extra calories.

When to Stop Working Out During Fasting. When fasting or working out, the most important thing to do is what your body is telling you because there is a large risk of reduction in the levels of your blood glucose. So if you have never done this before, do not register for a rigorous session that might involve maximum exertion of your heart. Do not overdo it. Overdoing it might make you feel light-headed or even lose consciousness due to a quick reduction in the levels of your blood glucose, and it is a scary situation when that happens.

A little bit of planning would be very beneficial. The most vital factor to consider while on an extended or intermittent fast is what your breakfast looks like and how it works well with your workout routine. It is vital to consume healthy fats, protein, organic fibers, and complex carbs during the eating period to sustain a healthy fast.

So, that's it. Rigorous, or less rigorous exercises, make sure to make suitable plans for your meals. Remember, the most important thing is to listen to your body. Do not engage in rigorous workouts if it's telling you not to do them. Throughout the fast, there will be a variation in your energy levels, from experiencing weakness and tiredness to experiencing energy bursts. Regardless of how energetic you feel, do not stress yourself. Rather, engage in calm, soothing yoga. Yoga is a gentle way of stretching out your muscles and engaging in mild exercises.

For some people, light stretches and yoga might be easy, and for others, it might be too rigorous. Do what makes you feel good and go from there.

The Significance of Sleep While Fasting

During water fasting, sleep is the next crucial thing after water intake. While sleeping, the body undergoes repair, restoration, detoxification, and metabolism. It also begins a growth phase where it stores up energy and the cells begin to grow. You're at an optimal state after a satisfactory 7-8 hours of sleep during fasting, and the rate of tissue renewal is increased while sleeping as opposed to being in an active state. Both sleep and fasting should complement each other to attain a better healthy body overall; therefore, a great advantage of fasting is its positive effect on sleep. Although during the fast, you may find it difficult to sleep as a result of the earlier energy surge, there will be a significant positive change in the pattern of sleep because of the regulation carried out by the body to bring back normalcy.

Professional Guidance During Water-Fasting

With proper medical supervision and adequate guidance, water fasting is an efficient and harmless way of assisting the body in self-restoration. However, like any other things that affect the body, there are some associated risks. For anyone that is considering undergoing a therapeutic fast, my advice would be to do this under the guidance of a certified IAHP expert who is trained in the process. The International Association of Hygienic Physicians consists of primary care doctors that are experts at supervising therapeutic fasts. Every approved member is a licensed osteopath, medical doctor or chiropractor, that has finalized at least a 6-month residency program at an authorized institution that is specialized in therapeutic fasts. Unlike in the past, fasting is now easily accessible due to the increase in the number of licensed professionals

Advantages of fasting under professional guidance. Maximum health is sustained when the body has adequate health requirements such as proper environment, psychology, and diet. If any of these requirements are inadequate, it affects your health. Most times, therapeutic fasting is an incredibly effective way of health recovery since it enables the body to produce an exceptional response to healing.

No other form of fasting can mimic the benefits of this way of fasting. Fasting, in a busy, noisy, or unsupportive surrounding will deprive the body of the chance to optimize the processes of self-restoration. Total rest is pertinent to optimize the beneficial effects of therapeutic fasting. Drinking juices exclusively or eating particular foods are essential as well. There are tremendous benefits both health and physiologically-wise when you consume these foods. However, this does not imply that the elimination diet, otherwise known as juice diet, is better than a straight water fast.

How A Chiropractor Will Help With The Fasting Process

Certain specialists in the health care sector concentrate on recognizing, and treating diseases that affect the junction between muscles and nerves, and they are very particular about curing these diseases by molding and sometimes, even altering the spinal cord. These specialists are called Chiropractors.

Chiropractors educate their patients on how to care for themselves by ergonomics, exercising, making user-friendly systems and other remedies to relieve back pain. Their main aim is to lessen the pain felt by patients and to increase their performance.

They believe that periodic fasting purges the body of harmful substances and causes the body to perform optimally.

There are certain criteria chiropractors take heed of during a fast;

First on the list of criteria is preventing death. Chiropractors expect side effects of fasting such as irritability, skin rashes, foul taste in the mouth, headaches, nausea and vomiting, unusual discharges from mucous membranes, postural hypertension and low back pain in the initial stage of fasting as a result of referral activity from kidney changes.

These professionals know that their patients undergo characteristic restorative crisis whereby persistent illnesses develop into short term illnesses and that it can be very distressing. Thus, their responsibility is to detect the boy's attempt to recover through a short term illness.

They are very mindful of carrying out the proper clinical supervision of their patients, after which they monitor the reaction of the body to the fast to determine the extent and severity of the therapy. To a great length, chiropractors monitor patient's activities like the food they eat, the time they sleep, and even as far as how susceptible they are to levels of stress.

Chiropractors can guarantee a risk-free experience, influencing the slightest reaction to water fasting (including hydration), as a result of the control they have over the patient's activities.

Chapter 9: How to Deal with Hunger During Water Fasting

It's crucial to note that starving yourself for fasting won't lead to death. This is pessimistic thoughts with fear works like a prophecy.

When you are a couple of minutes into a fast, and feeling hungry, telling yourself you can't do it, and the next meal you're going to eat dominates your mind, it's not going to take you anywhere.

Your body as a human has been transformed to control periods of fasting. Even when you come to think of it, there's no evolutionary logic attached to eating 3-5 meals per day. Naturally, we don't have anything like 3-5 sure meals on a daily. Too much availability of food only became possible in this new era.

Understand the Difference Between Psychological and Physical Hunger

Circadian clocks afford animals to predict daily events instead of ordinarily reacting to them. Also, the cells that create ghrelin possess circadian clocks that probably synchronize the expectation of food with metabolic cycles. In a nutshell, this means that eating a set of meals per day is trained and mastered behavior.

Most times we seem that we are hungry, we're not feeling true physiological or body hunger, rather what we're experiencing is psychological or head hunger. Immediately we notice this, then all it will take is to be disconnected from it until our system adapts to the fasting routine.

My Experience

In theory, fasting seems very easy. You could be thinking - yeah I will only avoid eating for some days and then continue with your meal afterward, but it goes beyond that. Personally, I have taken part in every type of fasting and failed several times. Every attempt I make looks pretty simple at the beginning. I used to be very excited concerning my latest plan that even the thought of eating never comes to my mind, I'd be so confident that I could bet on my success.

I'm committed at the starting of every fast, that I would choose to stick with one. Meaning it's not until 20hrs plus that the interest of the fast starts to depreciate, and I begin to lose the motivating spirit to keep going. However, now I understand that what kept me quitting was that I thought I would reach the initial slump, which is unavoidable because everyone fasting goes through it as well. To me seems as if my brain is testing me to know if this is really what I desire.

It will be obvious to you when you hit the slumping state because, at that point, you'll be asking yourself whether you're doing the right thing, the mind will randomly remind you to eat something. But if you can be able to defeat that urge, you'll be empowered to continue your fast. That slump should be seen as a battle, in which you must fight and win to accomplish your goal. Make sure you're prepared for it and also expect it.

Fasting isn't an easy task, The beginning might be interesting to you, but it becomes tougher as time progresses, to the extent that you'll feel like giving up and eating anything in the cupboard or even buying a pizza to sustain the moment. AVOID DOING IT.

Follow this advice to succeed. Do yourself a favor and be sure to practice these tips before giving up.

- Always expect hunger
- Draft a plan detailing your strategy when you begin to feel the hunger

Take Tea or Coffee Without Adding Sugar

Everyone knows that caffeine provides you with energy, but not everyone knows it's a potent appetite suppressant. Coffee/tea can be used to stop the urge to eat for the whole day. Drinking hot tea or coffee can help in making a person feel as if he or she has eaten. Also, the truth that you're drinking something tasty makes it feel a lot like a meal.

Here's the question, should you use milk or not?

When your aim of fasting is to shed weight, then adding a small quantity of milk to your drink is healthy while those who are fasting for religious reasons or cleansing could brew their drink without adding milk.

If you prefer to be very strict, consume it black, although it doesn't make so much difference. You could add a dash of milk (not more than 6ml) and still be in a fasted state.

- Caffeine in tea/coffee represses your appetite

- Adding milk won't stop your fast

Ensure You're Drinking Plenty of Water

Thirst can appear like hunger. It might seem as if you're starving, but in the real sense, you're dehydrating. During fasting, a lot of water is removed from your body. Consume 2-3 liters of water daily when fasting. Lethargy and headaches are notable signs of dehydration, so when you experience these during fasting, drink more and more water. But if you aren't feeling the thirst to drink enough water, it could be that you've gotten to balance of salt-to-water in your blood. To solve this problem, add a small pinch of pink Himalayan salt into your water. It will also contribute to your electrolytes too.

Water is wonderful as it makes you feel fulfilled, but don't over consume it. Drinking massive amounts of water frequently will do more harm to you than good. The idea is to drink water whenever you feel hungry because consuming water unnecessarily will only make you urinate frequently and this flushes out your electrolytes that may cause flu-like symptoms. Make sure to stick with 2-3 liters and space out your durational consumption, and you'll be okay.

- Drink it when hunger comes knocking
- 2-3 liters every day
- Spread the water intake throughout the entire day

Go to Bed

It's baffling to note that a lot of people don't know that sleeping equals fasting as well.

The evening is the peak time that most people will break their fast, including me. I'll abide by it every day, then when evening comes around, I give in and join my family during dinner. Whenever this happens, I see it as a failure in my part by writing off the week and starting anew on Monday of another week. The whole thing will want to repeat itself over and over again.

I have realized going to bed earlier would help me succeed that hard part, and waking up 8 hrs later it would've been the next morning. It's very hard to break your fast in the night if you follow this trick. Breaking your fast will make you feel bad the next day, rather than good, so try to sleep and see whether you'll still be hungry by morning.

It's advisable to begin your fast before going to bed, and using this strategy will make your first 8 hrs of fasting much easier and hunger-free.

- If you desire to give up when evening comes around, fight that urge off strongly

- Try to sleep whenever you're hungry at night

Remember that hunger comes in waves. It will pass.

Many people don't understand how long hunger takes because they're prompted to eat something whenever they get little feeling of hunger. They're always afraid of the word "hunger" and began to eat anytime their system churns with hunger. Those who are used to fasting know that if you endure a bit, the hunger will leave. Just put it in your mind you'll eat later because even feelings of hunger don't take more than 20 minutes or so, which starts to reduce as time passes.

Hunger is as a result of increased ghrelin. That is, ghrelin increases when you begin fasting, which leads to hunger. The increased levels of ghrelin don't remain permanent, meaning hunger reduces as fasting continues. During your weight loss journey ensure you also have this in mind. When the hiccups come around during that feeling of hunger remember to tell yourself: "This feeling of hunger in me will vanish soon" then move on with your fasting.

- Hunger pangs only stay for 20 minutes before it starts to vanish

- Your hormone ghrelin causes the feeling of hunger

- The level of ghrelin reduces during ketosis

Distract Yourself

Human beings tend to mistake boredom for hunger. We tend to eat whenever we're bored because it keeps us busy. I was ignorant of how much eating food took out of my time during the day until I began to fast. I use to think that only the time spent on a meal is only the time we took to eat, but it was wrong. Thinking of what to consume at breakfast, lunch, dinner and what we'll eat during those times takes out a considerable amount of time spent because we spend much time thinking about it before eventually eating it.

It doesn't make sense when we start fasting, and our mind is still preoccupied with food. This happens because we have our normal day wired out of habit to be around food. So much so that even when you're not hungry, your system still triggers you to consume something as you keep thinking about it throughout the day.

How do you fight this anomaly during fasting? Try to distract yourself.

Try to pamper yourself. Personal care during fasting is my favorite strategy to kill time. Although fasting is difficult, take some time out to reward yourself. Immerse yourself in the tub with Epsom salts and read or listen to an interesting book. Go out and get a good haircut. Take a spa day. You're going through something incredibly difficult, and you deserve to be pampered.

Be organized. Organizing or cleaning around the house is another great distraction you could follow. For me, I always try to make lists of things during my non-fasting days that I'll do while fasting.

There are always little things we need to do around our home, office, and so on. They seem always to bother you but haven't made time for them. Now is your chance to take care of those bothersome errands. You could empty the messy closet that you've been using for years to be cleaned, clean and rearrange your storage cupboard, clean the dishes and wash your car, or delve into other chores. Some distractions that come with physical involvement can be very effective and also give you a light workout too.

Indulge Yourself. There's absolutely nothing embarrassing in engaging in unproductive activities to help you pass through a fast state because using few hours to play is better than giving up to achieve your desired result due to boredom. Watch videos on YouTube, watch your desired TV program, play games, and more.

I resort to checking my email, replying to Twitter or Facebook messages, whenever I feel bored and hungry. Normally, I would've stopped myself from doing these as it's unproductive, but I believe that it's better to be unproductive than to fail my fast because I know my health matters!

It's not difficult to realize when it's boredom that you're suffering from and not hunger. When you notice this, try to play around for some minutes to push through. Once the hunger vanishes, you can start your work again.

Go out for a walk. Most times, leaving the house or office is very helpful in keeping you going when you feel like giving up. You could decide to go to the store and buy some sparkling water, or tea, go and visit a friend. Even getting up to walk around the house or work with no aim in mind helps too.

When I reach the point that I'm doing this, I try to remember that my aim is my overall health and well-being. I imagine how happy I will be after achieving my goal and how people will feel after seeing me lose weight. Thinking of this while fresh air cools my frayed nerves keeps me inspired to move on with my fast.

Focus. By using your brain power effectively, your mind will automatically ignore thinking of food. Try to learn new things and put them into practice immediately like learning a new language or even a new hobby. Personally, I throw myself into a book or something that needs my full attention.

Nevertheless, the higher level of adrenaline and orexin in your system will help you to be up-and-doing, meaning your brain can take-in educative information easily and comfortably. Put it into practice, and you'll be surprised at how useful you can be with that extra time you're not worried over what to eat.

- Those times that you think you're hungry not knowing you're only bored

- Delve into your normal routine and get rid of boredom

Flee from Places Where You Can Smell or See Food

This reason made me break a lot of my fasts in the beginning. As I move on with my fasting confidently, thinking nothing will be able to stop me, I accidentally smell delicious food from somewhere. That very next moment I'd go for that meal and start eating, knowing I won't be happy with myself for the next 20 minutes. I suffered from this problem for quite a while, and I also know that it will happen again. I began to wonder the reason why I couldn't hold myself back since I knew it wasn't hunger, but I kept falling to that little test. So what was it?

We're are programmed in a way that if we see or smell food, we start salivating to it. Immediately our digestive system opens for food intake, and our mouths began to water. Before we know it, our brain starts screaming at us to Eat! Eat!! Eat now!!!

It will take you a monk's discipline to resist eating food. Even if you don't, don't beat yourself up too much about it. The easiest and only way to avoid this is to stay away from hot food in those few days of your fast. As those days pass, you would be in ketosis and resisting won't be challenging any longer.

If you're the type that cooks for other people like yourself, make them understand that you're in your fasting days and can't cook for those periods. If that isn't possible, you could buy takeout food or schedule preparing a meal for them during your non-fasting days.

- Being close to food will make your body want to eat

- Resisting the urge to eat is incredibly difficult when your brain is pushing you to eat something

Meditate

You can remove yourself from feelings of hunger by practicing meditation. Push yourself far away from the urge to eat until that cravings disappear.

One other best idea to eliminate hunger or craving for food is to shift your focus. Whether you're fasting or not, meditation helps greatly to rid your head-space, but together with fasting, meditation and fasting enhance and synergize each other.

- You're free to meditate at any point in time

- For beginners, it's healthy to practice guided meditation

Remember Why You Started

Always remember that you engaged in fasting for a purpose, and not for the sake that you don't feel like eating. Try to write the reasons that made you go into fasting, daily. What's that thing you want to change by fasting? Are you fasting for personal reasons? And why?

Try to write down the reasons you're fasting after doing it today. Do it tomorrow as well, because most people easily forget their reasons for doing something. Make it a habit of reminding yourself daily by writing it down as many times as possible so that it will be imprinted in your brain.

From now on anytime your memory tells you to eat it will immediately ring in your head that you're fasting.

- So write those reasons down so you'll know them by heart

- Don't forget that it's only you who can personally end the fast

Habit Changes

Anyone who fasts to lose weight and yet doesn't make any habit/diet changes will gradually recover all the weight used up during the fasting period

If your goal for doing a water fast is to lose weight, ensure your first focus is to change your eating habits, then gradually proceed to water fasting via the previously explained methods. Upon returning to your usual self, stick to your changed diet habit.

Old habits vs. New habits – begins with:

- Staying away from animal products: All dairy products, eggs, and meat. You'll shed so much weight by doing this, and it'll make you look and feel a lot better.

- Along with every meal, eat a big serving of green leafy salad.

- Include one freshly extracted vegetable juice in your everyday routine.

- Also, in your everyday meal plan, include activated charcoal and alkaline water in your diet.

- Engage in one short water fast every week, or intermittent water fast every month, or 3-day extended water fast every three months.

Following these steps will help you ensure success in stopping the old habits and keeping the new habits.

Chapter 10: Frequently Asked Questions

Who can fast?

For a few conditions, fasting is not recommended. During a fast, fatty acids are required as a substitute energy source, but a small percentage of people do not possess the enzyme that is necessary to metabolize fatty acids as a result of an inborn error of metabolism. A prolonged duration of fasting is not advisable for this set of people. An expert can quickly identify this inborn error at the start of fasting.

Certain conditions are not favorable to fasting, and they include; Pregnancy, some forms of cancer, use of some medications, kidney and liver disorders, severe weakness, and starvation.

How to know when to fast?

Knowing when to fast is dependent on your current health status and what you plan to achieve by fasting. For most people, taking up a complete change in diet, participating in a realistic exercise plan, getting adequate sleep, and living in a somewhat hygienic environment will contribute to the conditions necessary for restoration, and sustenance of vital health. Fasting can be very instrumental in promoting recovery especially when one is finding it hard to change their diet and lifestyle. Fasting can help to defeat addictions to recreational drugs like nicotine, alcohol, and caffeine, and stimulants like salt, sugar by re-adjusting the nervous system's sensitivity. Fasting has helped people appreciate the crude, natural taste of good food as you hear testimonials talking about romaine lettuce's sweetness, an apple's fresh taste, and the unbelievably rich taste of baked potatoes even without butter, and sour cream.

Some decide to fast without the apparent evidence of disease with the knowledge that a total physiological reset will cause the body to renew itself and rid itself of toxins accumulated in tissues despite our attempts at living right.

How long can you water fast for without causing any harm?

Depending on your experience with water fasting, I'd advise a first timer not to water fast for more than three days (72 hours).

It has been agreed in the community of water fasting that even though one might have some experience with fasting, water fasting for more than three days is best done under close supervision by medical experts in a fasting retreat.

This is unarguably true as there are several reasons why the retreat makes fasting much easier; those reasons are:

- The availability of a medical expert on call to answer all your questions

- There are no interruptions by any activities from your daily routine.

- The retreat is filled with people of like minds, also keen on fasting

The expensive fee for the fasting retreat, and sometimes the unwillingness of patients used to the idea of pausing one's daily routine for a couple of weeks is the sole drawback of a fasting retreat.

How frequently do I have to water fast?

To rejuvenate the immune system, one should embark on a 3-day fast quarterly (that is, every 12 weeks, or every three months) or it can be one only once a year for 7-10 days to lower the frequency of cancer incidences to a large extent.

What kind of water do I drink?

It is possible for one to have a disproportion of electrolytes and lack of minerals, in this case, it is advisable to drink mineral water. You should also drink sparkling water and regular water.

Is tea allowed during a water fast?

Pure water fasting involves water exclusively. It is not harmful if you add tea to your water fast and it might be helpful because it provides natural nutrients. Drink only tea containing water and avoid milk.

What amount of weight is lost on a water fast?

Each person is different, and only your body can determine how much you will lose. It is recommended that losing weight using water fasting should be done with the guidance of a doctor and weight loss should not exceed 1.1 kg (or two and a half pounds) every week.

Is it possible for me to lose muscle?

The majority of muscle loss occurs in the first 3-4 days of fasting, so it is generally dependent on the way you fast. Once your body begins to produce ketones as an alternative source of energy to glucose, the body is said to be in ketosis, and this attempt to save protein is what leads to the loss of muscle, albeit fairly small.

What is ketosis?

After eating the food eaten is turned into glucose which gives energy to the brain, muscles and other parts of the body. Your body makes use of the leftover glucose and starts to breakdown fatty acids in the liver to manufacture ketones when you've not eaten. During a fast, ketones are another form of energy which the body uses competently- the brain, heart, cells loves ketones, and they like ketones better (the primary source of energy of the heart are fatty acids). Ketosis is a state where ketones are the only source of energy used by the body.

What is the difference between juice fasting and water fasting?

Water fasting limits your intake to water exclusively, and sometimes tea; whereas a juice fast allows fruit juices and various vegetables. If correctly done, juice fasting increases your energy levels and maintain your blood glucose. Otherwise, it might result in fluctuations levels of blood sugar, and this can be dangerous.

Can I do a juice fast instead?

The purpose of water fasting is attaining and sustaining ketosis quickly, as ketosis helps you enjoy the benefits sooner. Even though juice fasting is beneficial too, the probability of reaching deep ketosis, or even reaching ketosis at all is low because of the higher sugar-water content compare to the fiber content.

Because of that difference, water fasting and juice fasting are not similar in any way.

How many glasses of water should I drink daily?

In a day, a range of 9-13 cups of water is ideal. ABOUT 13 glasses of water and fluids equivalent to 3 liters are ideal for men, and 9 cups equal to 2.2 liters is ideal for women. You can drink pure water available or water that has been distilled or simply continue with the recommended intake with regular tap water.

Try not to drink it all at a go! You could fill three 1-liter jugs to monitor the volume you are drinking and try to break your drinking into smaller quantities for the day.

Make sure not to drink more than the advised quantity of water daily because it can cause health problems since it creates an imbalance of minerals and salt in the body.

Fight hunger spells. Tackle hunger pains by consuming 1-2 cups of water then relax or take a nap if you're able; the urge to eat will generally pass. Also, meditation and reading a book can help take your mind off it.

Can I be productive during a fast?

For the initial five days in a 10-days fast, you will not think about doing much, so the best you can do is rest throughout that period. After the five days, you will be without strength, and there will be low blood pressure (postural hypertension-being unable to stand up fast), but you will possibly be motivated to read, work, learn or do other things because while in ketosis you'll feel psychologically energized. If you cannot schedule five or more days of rest, begin with a three-day water fast over a weekend or for five days beginning from Thursday and finishing on a Monday.

Won't I gain back more weight after a fast since my rate of metabolism will reduce while I'm fasting and after the fast?

Our time our physiological needs causes alterations in metabolic rate. During vigorous activities, our metabolic rate fires up and during rest/sleep our the metabolic rate declines. From this time, during a fast our metabolic rate declines because there's a reduction in physiological requirements compared to times when one is carrying out their routine activities and eating. Metabolic rate increases to correlate with rising physiological needs when a person breaks a fast and returns to their previous activities.

During a fast, the assimilative and digestive capacity is altered. A fast brings about the repair of the digestive organs hence optimizing nutrients intake. Gaining or losing weight is merely dependent on the number of calories taken in compared to the number broken down.

Can IBS be cured by water fasting?

Usually, the initial recommendation for IBS is frequent meals and diet patterns, and this is the best piece of advice that people with IBS are given. Although there is no long-term, direct research concerning fasting for people with IBS, there may be some issues for them.

First, fasting; particularly in the absence of professional guidance, might lead to a lowered intake of some nutrients in the diet, resulting in a high risk of nutritional imbalances.

Secondly, there is a reduction in the content of food such as fiber and probiotics that are specific to the gut, and this might reduce the number of bacteria that are beneficial to the gut.

Can kidney stones result from water fasting?

There are disparities in the studies carried out on the prevalence of kidney stones, renal colic, and urinary stones while on a fast. The outcomes of research in the connection between fasting and urinary stones are different and, in some cases, might be conflicting. Most research suggests that an increase in the incidence of urinary stones is not connected to fasting but is as a result of weather changes, increase in temperature and increased humidity. So, if you have a higher risk of developing a kidney stone, rather than engaging in extended fasting, I advise intermittent fasting as a better option.

Can ulcers result from water fasting?

There is no proof that fasting causes ulcers in the small intestine and stomach. Digestion of food is enhanced by the acids that are secreted by the stomach, and these acids are also protective against microorganisms. Mucus is also produced to protect the lining of the small intestine and stomach. Ulcers are caused by sores that result from the acid in the stomach acting on a reduced or worn out mucus lining that can no longer protect body tissues. This might occur in the intestine or stomach and is known as gastric ulcer or peptic ulcer.

Stomach ulcers result from long-term H.pylori infection and a reduction in the protective mucus lining of the stomach. There is a reduction in the mucous when NSAIDs(nonsteroidal anti-inflammatory drugs) are used for a long time, since they inhibit inflammation, they also inhibit the production of mucus. It is doubtful that only fasting would result in ulcers, except in people with already existing gastritis and ulcers, it could aggravate the symptoms.

A lot of people suffering from ulcers are relieved after drinking or eating while pain associated with an ulcer is made worse by many foods. Therefore, an ulcer is caused by bacteria, probably with NSAID use and highly unlikely with fasting. Consult your doctor. If you are on a drug to manage your ulcer, fasting is probably not for you.

Is an enema advisable?

Avoid getting an enema (colon cleansing) while in a water fast. Although there is a misconception that an enema is essential, science has discovered no proof that it is beneficial, it might even be harmful to your health. Enemas can result in, cramping, vomiting and bloating.

Conclusion

I used to practice one-day water fasting weekly during my twenties, and it was an enlightening experience that I remember well. Over time, those one-day fasts became easier to do, and I always felt refreshed and renewed.

As time moved along and the older I got, I had stumbled across other ways to rid myself of toxins besides water fasting; such as the intake of cleansing herbs for my colon and complete body cleansing, routine raw vegan meals, occasional fasting from meals.

The processes such as repairing and detoxifying that happens while fasting also happens when a person is actively consuming meals. For people whose conditions are not getting better as quickly as they want it to or those that need a specific time of healing for resolution, a fast can be greatly beneficial. It is also important to note that it is a person's lifestyle after the fast that is the most crucial aspect of the fast. Fasting gives a fresh and renewed baseline to develop a flourishing body by regularly choosing to eat healthily and live right.

For detoxification, and other health benefits I still personally rely on short term and periodic water fasting over the course of a meal, a day, or even a few days.

Water fasting for more than three days needs detailed planning (before and after), self-education and also professional assistance as required.

Fasting can be an arduous ordeal, depending on one's health, emotional and mental state.

Hence, I recommend that before, during, and after a fast consider the physical advantages of the fast over your overall state of health. Knowing this will reduce the acute stress produced by those adverse effects which obviously does not boost your health and make you feel better.

Water fasting is one of the most natural diets on earth if you follow the most crucial rule of consuming adequate water throughout the fast and some other additional tips like not standing up too fast.

Remember that that water fasting may be simple does not make it easy.

Other diets do not genuinely remove hunger, and this is the significant advantage that water fasting has over diets – if you water fast properly hunger is completely eliminated.

Reference

1. Zimmer, C. (2019). Self-Destructive Behavior in Cells May Hold Key to a Longer Life. Retrieved from https://www.nytimes.com/2009/10/06/science/06cell.html?pagewanted=all&_r=1

2. Ohsumi, Y. (2013). Historical landmarks of autophagy research. Cell Research, 24(1), 9-23. doi: 10.1038/cr.2013.169

3. Autophagy 101: How Intermittent Fasting Could Help Us Age Slowly. (2019). Retrieved from https://thechalkboardmag.com/what-is-autophagy-intermittent-fasting-process

4. Madeo, F., Zimmermann, A., Maiuri, M., & Kroemer, G. (2015). Essential role for autophagy in life span extension. Journal Of Clinical Investigation, 125(1), 85-93. doi: 10.1172/jci73946

5. Shetty, A., Kodali, M., Upadhya, R., & Madhu, L. (2018). Emerging Anti-Aging Strategies - Scientific Basis and Efficacy. Aging And Disease, 9(6), 1165. doi: 10.14336/ad.2018.1026

6. Mizushima, N., Yoshimori, T., & Ohsumi, Y. (2011). The Role of Atg Proteins in Autophagosome Formation. Annual Review Of Cell And Developmental Biology, 27(1), 107-132. doi: 10.1146/annurev-cellbio-092910-154005

7. Mizushima, N., Ohsumi, Y., & Yoshimori, T. (2002). Autophagosome Formation in Mammalian Cells. Cell Structure And Function, 27(6), 421-429. doi: 10.1247/csf.27.421

8. Castro-Obregon, S. (2019). Lysosomes, Autophagy | Learn Science at Scitable. Retrieved from https://www.nature.com/scitable/topicpage/the-discovery-of-lysosomes-and-autophagy-14199828

9. Bandyopadhyay, U., Kaushik, S., Varticovski, L., & Cuervo, A. (2008). The Chaperone-Mediated Autophagy Receptor Organizes in Dynamic Protein Complexes at the Lysosomal Membrane. Molecular And Cellular Biology, 28(18), 5747-5763. doi: 10.1128/mcb.02070-07

10. Gump, J., & Thorburn, A. (2011). Autophagy and apoptosis: what is the connection?. Trends In Cell Biology, 21(7), 387-392. doi: 10.1016/j.tcb.2011.03.007

11. Alirezaei, M., Kemball, C., Flynn, C., Wood, M., Whitton, J., & Kiosses, W. (2010). Short-term fasting induces profound neuronal autophagy. Autophagy, 6(6), 702-710. doi: 10.4161/auto.6.6.12376

12. He, C., Sumpter, Jr., R., & Levine, B. (2012). Exercise induces autophagy in peripheral tissues and in the brain. Autophagy, 8(10), 1548-1551. doi: 10.4161/auto.21327

13. Land, S. (2019). Mistruths and Lies About Autophagy. Retrieved from

https://siimland.com/mistruths-and-lies-about-autophagy/

14. Westerterp, K. (2004). Nutrition & Metabolism, 1(1), 5. doi: 10.1186/1743-7075-1-5

15. Bellisle F, e. (2019). Meal frequency and energy balance. - PubMed - NCBI. Retrieved from https://www.ncbi.nlm.nih.gov/pubmed/9155494

16. Smeets, A., & Westerterp-Plantenga, M. (2007). Acute effects on metabolism and appetite profile of one meal difference in the lower range of meal frequency. British Journal Of Nutrition, 99(06). doi: 10.1017/s0007114507877646

17. Leidy, H., Armstrong, C., Tang, M., Mattes, R., & Campbell, W. (2010). The Influence of Higher Protein Intake and Greater Eating Frequency on Appetite Control in Overweight and Obese Men. Obesity, 18(9), 1725-1732. doi: 10.1038/oby.2010.45

18. SPEECHLY, D., & BUFFENSTEIN, R. (1999). Greater Appetite Control Associated with an Increased Frequency of Eating in Lean Males. Appetite, 33(3), 285-297. doi: 10.1006/appe.1999.0265

19. Jon Schoenfeld, B., Albert Aragon, A., & Krieger, J. (2015). Effects of meal frequency on weight loss and body composition: a meta-analysis. Nutrition Reviews, 73(2), 69-82. doi: 10.1093/nutrit/nuu017

20. Cameron, J., Cyr, M., & Doucet, É. (2009). Increased meal frequency does not promote greater weight loss in subjects who were prescribed an 8-week equi-energetic energy-restricted diet. British Journal Of Nutrition, 1. doi: 10.1017/s0007114509992984

21. Alirezaei, M., Kemball, C., Flynn, C., Wood, M., Whitton, J., & Kiosses, W. (2010). Short-term fasting induces profound neuronal autophagy. Autophagy, 6(6), 702-710. doi: 10.4161/auto.6.6.12376

22. Koopman, K., Caan, M., Nederveen, A., Pels, A., Ackermans, M., & Fliers, E. et al. (2014). Hypercaloric diets with increased meal frequency, but not meal size, increase intrahepatic triglycerides: A randomized controlled trial. Hepatology, 60(2), 545-553. doi: 10.1002/hep.27149

23. de Verdier, M., & Longnecker, M. (1992). Eating frequency—a neglected risk factor for colon cancer?. Cancer Causes & Control, 3(1), 77-81. doi: 10.1007/bf00051916

24. Heilbronn, L., Smith, S., Martin, C., Anton, S., & Ravussin, E. (2005). Alternate-day fasting in nonobese subjects: effects on body weight, body composition, and energy metabolism. The American Journal Of Clinical Nutrition, 81(1), 69-73. doi: 10.1093/ajcn/81.1.69

25. Arnal, M., Mosoni, L., Boirie, Y., Houlier, M., Morin, L., & Verdier, E. et al. (1999). Protein pulse feeding improves protein retention in elderly women. The American Journal Of

Clinical Nutrition, 69(6), 1202-1208. doi: 10.1093/ajcn/69.6.1202

26. Varady, K. (2011). Intermittent versus daily calorie restriction: which diet regimen is more effective for weight loss?. Obesity Reviews, 12(7), e593-e601. doi: 10.1111/j.1467-789x.2011.00873.x

27. Stote, K., Baer, D., Spears, K., Paul, D., Harris, G., & Rumpler, W. et al. (2007). A controlled trial of reduced meal frequency without caloric restriction in healthy, normal-weight, middle-aged adults. The American Journal Of Clinical Nutrition, 85(4), 981-988. doi: 10.1093/ajcn/85.4.981

28. Barnosky, A., Hoddy, K., Unterman, T., & Varady, K. (2014). Intermittent fasting vs daily calorie restriction for type 2 diabetes prevention: a review of human findings. Translational Research, 164(4), 302-311. doi: 10.1016/j.trsl.2014.05.013

29. 5 Day Water Fast: What to Expect on the Healing Journey - DrJockers.com. (2019). Retrieved

from https://drjockers.com/water-fast/

30. Water Fasting: 12 Strategies to Prepare Properly - DrJockers.com. (2019). Retrieved from https://drjockers.com/water-fasting/

31. Cheng, C., Adams, G., Perin, L., Wei, M., Zhou, X., & Lam, B. et al. (2014). Prolonged Fasting Reduces IGF-1/PKA to Promote Hematopoietic-Stem-Cell-Based Regeneration and Reverse Immunosuppression. Cell Stem Cell, 14(6), 810-823. doi: 10.1016/j.stem.2014.04.014

32. Paoli, A. (2014). Ketogenic Diet for Obesity: Friend or Foe?. International Journal Of Environmental Research And Public Health, 11(2), 2092-2107. doi: 10.3390/ijerph110202092

33. Takagi, A., Kume, S., Maegawa, H., & Uzu, T. (2016). Emerging role of mammalian autophagy in ketogenesis to overcome starvation. Autophagy,

12(4), 709-710. doi: 10.1080/15548627.2016.1151597

34. Varady, K., Bhutani, S., Church, E., & Klempel, M. (2009). Short-term modified alternate-day fasting: a novel dietary strategy for weight loss and cardioprotection in obese adults. The American Journal Of Clinical Nutrition, 90(5), 1138-1143. doi: 10.3945/ajcn.2009.28380

35. Heilbronn, L., Smith, S., Martin, C., Anton, S., & Ravussin, E. (2005). Alternate-day fasting in nonobese subjects: effects on body weight, body composition, and energy metabolism. The American Journal Of Clinical Nutrition, 81(1), 69-73. doi: 10.1093/ajcn/81.1.69

36. Cava, E., Yeat, N., & Mittendorfer, B. (2017). Preserving Healthy Muscle during Weight Loss. Advances In Nutrition: An International Review Journal, 8(3), 511-519. doi: 10.3945/an.116.014506

37. Leidy, H., Mattes, R., & Campbell, W. (2007). Effects of Acute and Chronic

Protein Intake on Metabolism, Appetite, and Ghrelin During Weight Loss*. Obesity, 15(5), 1215-1225. doi: 10.1038/oby.2007.143

Notes

[←1]

Ohsumi, Y. (2013). Historical landmarks of autophagy research. *Cell Research*, *24*(1), 9-23. doi: 10.1038/cr.2013.169

[←2]

Autophagy 101: How Intermittent Fasting Could Help Us Age Slowly. (2019). Retrieved from https://thechalkboardmag.com/what-is-autophagy-intermittent-fasting-process

[←3]

Mizushima, N., Yoshimori, T., & Ohsumi, Y. (2011). The Role of Atg Proteins in Autophagosome Formation. *Annual Review Of Cell And Developmental Biology*, 27(1), 107-132. doi: 10.1146/annurev-cellbio-092910-154005

[←4]

Mizushima, N., Ohsumi, Y., & Yoshimori, T. (2002). Autophagosome Formation in Mammalian Cells. Cell Structure And Function, 27(6), 421-429. doi: 10.1247/csf.27.421

[←5]

Castro-Obregon, S. (2019). Lysosomes, Autophagy | Learn Science at Scitable. Retrieved from https://www.nature.com/scitable/topicpage/the-discovery-of-lysosomes-and-autophagy-14199828

[←6]

Bandyopadhyay, U., Kaushik, S., Varticovski, L., & Cuervo, A. (2008). The Chaperone-Mediated Autophagy Receptor Organizes in Dynamic Protein Complexes at the Lysosomal Membrane. *Molecular And Cellular Biology*, *28*(18), 5747-5763. doi: 10.1128/mcb.02070-07

[←7]

Gump, J., & Thorburn, A. (2011). Autophagy and apoptosis: what is the connection?. *Trends In Cell Biology*, *21*(7), 387-392. doi: 10.1016/j.tcb.2011.03.007

[←8]

Alirezaei, M., Kemball, C., Flynn, C., Wood, M., Whitton, J., & Kiosses, W. (2010). Short-term fasting induces profound neuronal autophagy. *Autophagy*, *6*(6), 702-710. doi: 10.4161/auto.6.6.12376

[←9]

He, C., Sumpter, Jr., R., & Levine, B. (2012). Exercise induces autophagy in peripheral tissues and in the brain. *Autophagy*, *8*(10), 1548-1551. doi: 10.4161/auto.21327

[←10]

Land, S. (2019). Mistruths and Lies About Autophagy. Retrieved from https://siimland.com/mistruths-and-lies-about-autophagy/

[←11]

Westerterp, K. (2004). *Nutrition & Metabolism*, *1*(1), 5. doi: 10.1186/1743-7075-1-5

[←12]

Bellisle F, e. (2019). Meal frequency and energy balance. - PubMed - NCBI. Retrieved from https://www.ncbi.nlm.nih.gov/pubmed/9155494

[←13]

Smeets, A., & Westerterp-Plantenga, M. (2007). Acute effects on metabolism and appetite profile of one meal difference in the lower range of meal frequency. *British Journal Of Nutrition*, *99*(06). doi: 10.1017/s0007114507877646

[←14]

Leidy, H., Armstrong, C., Tang, M., Mattes, R., & Campbell, W. (2010). The Influence of Higher Protein Intake and Greater Eating Frequency on Appetite Control in Overweight and Obese Men. *Obesity*, *18*(9), 1725-1732. doi: 10.1038/oby.2010.45

[←15]

SPEECHLY, D., & BUFFENSTEIN, R. (1999). Greater Appetite Control Associated with an Increased Frequency of Eating in Lean Males. *Appetite, 33*(3), 285-297. doi: 10.1006/appe.1999.0265

[←16]

Jon Schoenfeld, B., Albert Aragon, A., & Krieger, J. (2015). Effects of meal frequency on weight loss and body composition: a meta-analysis. *Nutrition Reviews*, 73(2), 69-82. doi: 10.1093/nutrit/nuu017

[←17]

Cameron, J., Cyr, M., & Doucet, É. (2009). Increased meal frequency does not promote greater weight loss in subjects who were prescribed an 8-week equi-energetic energy-restricted diet. *British Journal Of Nutrition*, 1. doi: 10.1017/s0007114509992984

[←18]

Alirezaei, M., Kemball, C., Flynn, C., Wood, M., Whitton, J., & Kiosses, W. (2010). Short-term fasting induces profound neuronal autophagy. *Autophagy, 6*(6), 702-710. doi: 10.4161/auto.6.6.12376

[←19]

Koopman, K., Caan, M., Nederveen, A., Pels, A., Ackermans, M., & Fliers, E. et al. (2014). Hypercaloric diets with increased meal frequency, but not meal size, increase intrahepatic triglycerides: A randomized controlled trial. *Hepatology*, *60*(2), 545-553. doi: 10.1002/hep.27149

[←20]

de Verdier, M., & Longnecker, M. (1992). Eating frequency—a neglected risk factor for colon cancer?. *Cancer Causes & Control*, *3*(1), 77-81. doi: 10.1007/bf00051916

[←21]

Heilbronn, L., Smith, S., Martin, C., Anton, S., & Ravussin, E. (2005). Alternate-day fasting in nonobese subjects: effects on body weight, body composition, and energy metabolism. *The American Journal Of Clinical Nutrition*, *81*(1), 69-73. doi: 10.1093/ajcn/81.1.69

[←22]

Arnal, M., Mosoni, L., Boirie, Y., Houlier, M., Morin, L., & Verdier, E. et al. (1999). Protein pulse feeding improves protein retention in elderly women. *The American Journal Of Clinical Nutrition*, *69*(6), 1202-1208. doi: 10.1093/ajcn/69.6.1202

[←23]

Varady, K. (2011). Intermittent versus daily calorie restriction: which diet regimen is more effective for weight loss?. *Obesity Reviews*, *12*(7), e593-e601. doi: 10.1111/j.1467-789x.2011.00873.x

[←24]

Stote, K., Baer, D., Spears, K., Paul, D., Harris, G., & Rumpler, W. et al. (2007). A controlled trial of reduced meal frequency without caloric restriction in healthy, normal-weight, middle-aged adults. *The American Journal Of Clinical Nutrition*, *85*(4), 981-988. doi: 10.1093/ajcn/85.4.981

[←25]

Barnosky, A., Hoddy, K., Unterman, T., & Varady, K. (2014). Intermittent fasting vs daily calorie restriction for type 2 diabetes prevention: a review of human findings. *Translational Research*, *164*(4), 302-311. doi: 10.1016/j.trsl.2014.05.013

[←26]

5 Day Water Fast: What to Expect on the Healing Journey - DrJockers.com. (2019). Retrieved from https://drjockers.com/water-fast/

[←27]

Water Fasting: 12 Strategies to Prepare Properly - DrJockers.com. (2019). Retrieved from https://drjockers.com/water-fasting/

[←28]

Cheng, C., Adams, G., Perin, L., Wei, M., Zhou, X., & Lam, B. et al. (2014). Prolonged Fasting Reduces IGF-1/PKA to Promote Hematopoietic-Stem-Cell-Based Regeneration and Reverse Immunosuppression. *Cell Stem Cell*, *14*(6), 810-823. doi: 10.1016/j.stem.2014.04.014

[←29]

Paoli, A. (2014). Ketogenic Diet for Obesity: Friend or Foe?. *International Journal Of Environmental Research And Public Health*, *11*(2), 2092-2107. doi: 10.3390/ijerph110202092

[←30]

Takagi, A., Kume, S., Maegawa, H., & Uzu, T. (2016). Emerging role of mammalian autophagy in ketogenesis to overcome starvation. *Autophagy*, *12*(4), 709-710. doi: 10.1080/15548627.2016.1151597

[←31]

Varady, K., Bhutani, S., Church, E., & Klempel, M. (2009). Short-term modified alternate-day fasting: a novel dietary strategy for weight loss and cardioprotection in obese adults. *The American Journal Of Clinical Nutrition*, *90*(5), 1138-1143. doi: 10.3945/ajcn.2009.28380

[←32]

Heilbronn, L., Smith, S., Martin, C., Anton, S., & Ravussin, E. (2005). Alternate-day fasting in nonobese subjects: effects on body weight, body composition, and energy metabolism. The American Journal Of Clinical Nutrition, 81(1), 69-73. doi: 10.1093/ajcn/81.1.69

[←33]

Cava, E., Yeat, N., & Mittendorfer, B. (2017). Preserving Healthy Muscle during Weight Loss. *Advances In Nutrition: An International Review Journal*, 8(3), 511-519. doi: 10.3945/an.116.014506

[←34]

Leidy, H., Mattes, R., & Campbell, W. (2007). Effects of Acute and Chronic Protein Intake on Metabolism, Appetite, and Ghrelin During Weight Loss*. *Obesity*, *15*(5), 1215-1225. doi: 10.1038/oby.2007.143

www.ingramcontent.com/pod-product-compliance
Lightning Source LLC
Chambersburg PA
CBHW031137020426
42333CB00013B/417